PARA-MEDIC

<u>War & Peace</u>
<u>Dave Benny Bentley</u>

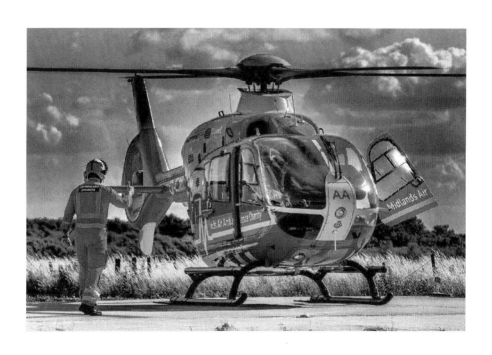

DAVE BENTLEY

PARA-MEDIC
WAR & PEACE
Dave Benny Bentley

Copyright © 2021 David Bentley

Authors Note

This is a true account of my story, the views and opinions expressed in this

Book are solely that of the author, and have not been endorsed by the MOD, NHS

Ambulances Trust's or the Midlands Air Ambulance Charity. Where necessary a number

Of names, dates and place names have been changed to protect people's identities and

obscure sensitive information. The medical contents written in this book should not be

treated as medical advice. For medical advice please consult your Doctor.

CONTENTS

My Story

Rhoda, Logan, George and Jude
You are my world

Dave "Benny" Bentley
A true story of a British Soldier that later became an NHS Paramedic, his experiences on what it was like fighting on 2 hugely different front lines

Prologue:

My name is Dave Bentley, I'd like everyone who is reading this, to know that I have had to fight many battles, physically and mentally. By writing this book, I am hoping that it may give, insight and direction to others, who may not have had the best of starts in life, empower them to go on to help others, not struggle with their own thoughts and demons and take a good path in life.

This book will take you on a journey through the eyes of a naughty young lad who joined the Army for adventure, the wars he fought both physically and mentally whilst in Iraq and Afghanistan as a British Soldier, and the situations he found himself in. It will touch on very special people that he met through the years and from there, move on from the military and focus on his experiences, the lives he saved and the lives he couldn't save as an NHS Paramedic, on a very different front line back at home.

This will be "a cards on the table" account of my career so far and I will try my best to explain all aspects of the journey and experiences that I have collected over the years. You will get a real feeling of what it was like for me and many others in my position. On two vastly different front lines.

THE PEGASUS PRAYER

O Lord, the everlasting God, Creator of the ends of the earth: You give the stallion his strength; his valour in war; he fears not the foe and leaps in the van of battle. Grant, also, that we may be courageous in conduct, chivalrous in conflict, just in all our words and deeds, humble, as we walk in your presence O God. For you promised of old that, as we trust in You, our strength will be renewed, we shall rise up on wings, we shall go forward and not grow weary, march and not be faint, through Jesus Christ out Lord, Amen.

THE PEGASUS ETHOS

As British Airborne soldiers we place the mission, and our comrades, before ourselves. Our bravery is founded upon determination, endurance, and selflessness. We are supremely disciplined and that discipline is primarily self-imposed. We take pride in being part of an elite, and we understand our responsibility to strive for the highest standards of achievement, turn-out and attitude. We wear Pegasus with humility, recognising our obligation never to demean or diminish the value of others. We are a compassionate friend, but a ferocious enemy. In battle, in barracks, and at home, we always do the right thing.

INTRODUCTION

I was born at New Cross Hospital, Wolverhampton at 21:00 on the 30th of May 1984. There was not much was happening around the world at this time, here I was!

Eight pound ten on the scales "fair play mom" and all was good. My Dad is called Andrew, I've only ever known him as Ben, who was a ground-worker and my mom is called Glennis who was working as a care assistant in a nursing home, they were, and are still, the greatest parents anyone could ever wish for.

I, along with my younger brother Drew, would put them to the test..........

"Dave, get up there and grab it "
This was my 12-year-old brother Drew, egging me on to climb up the edge of a railway bank, lie in wait and ambush a slow-passing container train for the prized flashing light on the last carriage of the train. As I remember my Dad's shed had at least 4 or 5 of these in there. I had to time it right, and just as the last trailer went passed I would sprint alongside the train, pull the white flashing box out of the bracket and lift it up to the sky, like I had just lifted the World Cup trophy. It used to give me a real buzz, no thought of the consequences of getting hurt, or not thinking about the trouble I could get into, this was living on the edge.

I always had this adventurous nature, always wanting to explore, climb trees, swim, and skim stones like a lot of us used to do. How different now with the invention of iPads, the internet and suchlike?

Back as a young lad, I would go out for hours and hours and only return home when the streetlights came on, usually starving or in trouble with the law. As you may be thinking, I said hours and hours, mostly during school hours. In truth, I was not there a lot.

CHAPTER 1

The Younger years

I attended Great Wyrley High School, which is now a Performing Arts College. I'll be honest, I did not enjoy school, not being a morning person. As a young lad, I used to put my uniform on the night before, so I could just roll out of my pit and walk up the road ready for class.

I was a skinny youth with that bowl head hair cut that we all used to have and must have always appeared scruffy and unkempt. I used to go to school purely to see my friends and have a scrap, I loved fighting! I reckon it must have been in the genes, as so did my Dad. He was like a Bulldog, standing at five feet eight inches tall and he was as wide as a brick shit house. I think I just wanted to be like him.

This was until this one moment, my uncle Paul gripped me at a family meal:

"you need to sort your shit out lad, you're good at sport, but shite at everything else" he hissed at me, and he was right.

Uncle Paul had just finished serving 23 years in the British Army as a Warrant officer 2 (WO2). He was tall, athletic, and well groomed. I looked up to him like a God. This was when I was about 14 years old, and from that moment, I knew what I wanted to do... I wanted to be a soldier..........

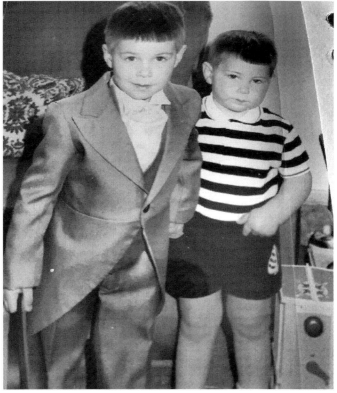

(Me left brother Drew right)

Before I could even consider joining the Army, I had to finish school. I hated it. The only thing I was any good at was sport, namely Rugby. I started playing Rugby when I was about 10 years old and it was my saviour. I loved every aspect of it, the teamwork, the tackles, the running, and the kicking. I was in my element every time I was anywhere near the game.

Rugby stopped me getting into trouble at school. I remember the day my PE teacher Mr Archbold said in his thick Geordie accent-

"Bentley you're not going to achieve anything with your written studies, but just maybe we can help you out with the physical stuff".

Mr Archbold and Mr Shiston were fantastic role models for me,

I think they knew I wasn't a bad lad, in fact I was very respect-ful as my parents had raised me to be, but I had this natural aggression that desperately needed channelling. They helped me achieve this through sport. They made me captain of the school team and gave me the opportunity to be selected for the county side, which, to this day, I am grateful for.

Without their intervention during my time at school, I would not have the grades or sport to guide me and would have been on a one-way track to a life behind bars, I think.

Leaving school, I had no GCSEs whatsoever; so, you may be thinking what the point was going? As the teachers kept on tell-ing me,

"Bentley, you have the potential to achieve",
However, I would rather be using my body instead of my brain.

So, I went and worked with my dad, when I was not at school. He was a landscaper who did driveways, patios, fencing and other bits. For me, this was great as I loved getting dirty, using tools, carrying and lifting stuff. A bonus was getting my body out for the ladies.

My Dad was a grafter, up early in the morning and home late at night, covered in mud everyday just to put some food on the table. I could tell he hated the work and was slowly falling to bits himself.

I remember him saying to me one day,

"I don't want this for you and your brother, get in that Army, get a trade and live the good life".

I will always remember this, and I always wanted to make him proud, and I still do....

I was now a spotty, skinny 16-year-old, who despite my best efforts, had had scrapes and dealings with the police, dis-covered beer and crazy women. I needed to get out of Wolver-hampton, get off to the Army Careers Office for myself.

The day came where I had to attend The British Army Recruit-ment interview at the Careers Office located in Queen's street in

Wolverhampton. To be blunt, I was shitting myself.

That morning I could not eat, I had to go to the toilet multiple times, and this was all from me: "Billy Big Balls" - thinking I am a rock-hard rugby player with all the minerals. Time to switch on and become a man! I dressed up smartly, shaved off the extraordinarily little crop of hair I had on my spotty chin, put some gel in my hair and slapped on the Joop. I was ready.

I got off the train wearing my blue Webster's suit and my highly polished shoes that my dad did for me, before he shot off to work that morning. I approached my target location. By this time, the nausea was immense and all the cockiness of a sixteen-year-old, know-it-all had gone. The doubts rushed at me from all sides and I was thinking up what excuses I could give my mom and dad to explain why it had been cancelled.

I got to the door and grabbed hold of my balls and said, "fuck it, let's go".

As I stepped through the massive red doors and before I could even take a deep breath in, I was met by-

"what the fuck is that on your head?"

My arse completely dropped out and I just didn't know what to do!

Now, why could this massive, hard-as-nails looking recruitment sergeant be shouting at me? Then I clicked! I had been on a rugby tour the week before and my hair still had blonde highlights in. Why I did not shave it all off before I went in is beyond me now, so we were off to a great start!

Following this fright of my life, I was invited into an office and was told to "sit down and I will deal with you in a minute" so I did as I was told. A couple of minutes passed, and as I glanced around, this same sergeant was staring right at me through the glass door and had clearly been doing it for some time, was I intimidated? - yes! Did I want my mom? Yes!!

I mentioned earlier that rugby was my saviour and this was a prime example when the sergeant asks, "right come on then, what the fuck is that all about on your head?"

In a squeaky voice I said, "what the blonde?"

He replied, "yes the fucking blonde, and its sergeant".

I explained that the week before I was on a rugby tour down south in Paignton. It was at that point you could see something change in his eyes and posture.

"A rugby player eh? Well, that's ok then let us get started".

From this moment I relaxed into the interview and we had a great chat around rugby, my local club Willenhall, to me representing Staffordshire county. He explained that if you play sport in the Army, you are well looked after and better fed, which was music to my ears. I love my grub. Once I settled down and relaxed a bit I started to look at him more, his uniform was smart, he had tattoos down his arms, and I wanted a piece of the action, had I of bottled it at the door, I can only imagine what sort of life I would have had now. So, my first piece of advice to you all is "be bold" and have a go, what is the worst that can happen?

"Success is not final; failure is not fatal: it is the courage to continue that counts" (Winston Churchill)

CHAPTER 2

<u>British Army Selection</u>

So, I passed my first interview at the Careers Office, the next stage was to attend a two-day selection at ATC Lichfield, where all the candidates would be put through their paces physically to see if they were eligible to gain entry into the British Army. I was more up for this and confident that I would do well, as it was the physical side, that appealed to me. As I mentioned earlier, I loved playing rugby and grafting with my dad, so I should be in my element.

I jumped on the train at Landywood station, waved good-bye to my mom, who was stood on the platform, and was crying. I thought she would be happy to have two days away from me, so I set off. I arrived at Lichfield train station, along with many other young lads, from all backgrounds, all of whom were dressed smartly. We all had a nervous aura around us. No one was talking, mixing, or making any eye contact with anyone else, it was a very eerie feeling. Nonetheless I thought let's have a go and do my mom and dad proud.

"Right, all of you who are here for British Army Selection, form up in three ranks so we can check you off. "

I was thinking - three ranks, what is all that about?

A corporal sorted us out, checked our names off the list and ordered us to jump on the back of a four tonner, (a big green lorry, with a swing tailgate) if any of you lucky people have ever got to travel in the back of one, you will understand that they are not built for comfort, especially if you get a middle seat. If you hit a bump, the seats move in different directions, clamp on to your arse and you get a bite which is worse than you would get from a Great White Shark! Okay, it is a slight exaggeration, but you get the gist!

We arrived at the camp, jumped of the trucks, and were then quickly directed to the stores to collect our bedding for the next two days. I was thinking fresh sheets, nice duvet. How wrong was I? This would be our first experience of itchy blankets.

We were put into the accommodation and that is the first time that we started to interact with each other, all trying to put a brave face on and help each other out. It felt strange to be there but quite relaxed at the same time. I thought there would be a lot of shouting and bawling in our young faces, but none of that, obviously this was the selection process, and the fun and games would come later.

During those two days we were put through various physical tests. We had to run a mile and half, pass strength tests, and then complete a medical. I was naïve to believe this would be the hardest part, well thankfully not.............

First, I had a sit down with a nice lady who asked me a few medical questions. Have I ever had Asthma? broke any bones? Just the normal generic questions you would get for a medical in any other job. I had my blood pressure taken, temperature and pulse and all seemed good. I moved on to the next part of the medical and waited to be seen by a doctor. Sitting patiently outside, ready to be called in, a youth shot out the door in front of me and with a surprised look on his face said to me.

"He's just grabbed me balls!!!"

I burst out laughing but then quickly realised it was my go next!

"Bentley!"

This was the moment and I stepped in for my assessment.

I was happy to report that it was a male doctor assessing me. As you can imagine at 16 years old, if it was a female in my case, things may be a little different. He asked me to strip down to my shreddies and perform a few movements, touch my toes, balance on one leg, cover your left eye, read the bottom letters etc which was a breeze. The next bit though was the most uncomfortable moment for me to date.

"Please can you drop your underpants?", I am going to assess your genitals."

I thought - if this is what the military will be like, I am not so sure if I want in. Anyway, in for penny and all that! I lowered my boxers and he proceeded to check my undercarriage, like rolling a couple of plums round in his hand. After an awkward minute or so he said I was good to go and that was the end of my medical. Phew!!

All done, the two days were quickly over, I did not know at this stage if I had passed or not but felt confident that I had done enough. Physically I was up there with the best but would soon learn my fate.

I Passed with flying colours! I was physically fit enough to gain entry into the British Army, I was ecstatic. The next step now was for me to attempt the BARB Test, an online programme at the careers office to see if I was bright enough to get a trade as my dad asked.

The BARB test (British Army Recruit Battery) Test is a psychometric test used by the Army to assess potential recruits to decide whether they are suitable for service and for what roles they are suitable for.

Looking back now, I am sure I could have smashed the test, but as I did not do well at school in the academic studies. I struggled with the test. I scored lower than I even thought possible, this ruled me out of getting a trade like engineering or medical, like I had hoped for.

The recruitment sergeant seemed really pleased.

"Why the long face?" he asked me.

I replied, I wanted a trade and make my dad proud. He put his arm on my shoulder and said.

"Look son I did the same and I wouldn't have had it any other way. You need to join the Paras!"

I never had even heard of 'The Paras' as I looked at him again with his Maroon Beret and Parachute wings on his right arm, he looked the dog's bollocks. I would have done anything he told me at that point.

He was obviously very proud of his unit as he said to me again.

"Men will want to be you, and women will hang off you like fruit bats"

So that was it, I decided I was going to be a Paratrooper.

CHAPTER 3

My Oath and the AFC

"I David George Bentley, swear by Almighty God that I will be faithful and bear true allegiance to Her Majesty Queen Elizabeth II, her heirs and successors and that I will as in duty bound honestly and faithfully defend Her Majesty, her heirs and successors in person, crown and dignity against all enemies and will observe and obey all orders of Her Majesty, her heirs and successors and of the generals and officers set over me".

Wow, I have just taken my Oath of Allegiance at Wolverhampton Civic Centre and made a promise to God, in front of my family. This was a massive moment in my young life at sixteen years of age, I was going to be part of the biggest family I would know. I am now a Soldier in the British Army.

AFC Harrogate (Army Foundation College) As I was sixteen unbelievably, I could not join the Army without permission from my mom and dad, quite ironically, we all had to sign on that dotted line. We set out from my forever home in Cheslyn Hay, near Wolverhampton in the West Midlands up the motorway until we reached our destination on Penny Pot Lane, North Yorkshire. This would be my new home for the next year. We parked up, we. grabbed my kit and made our way to the gym where military instructors met us. I was told at this moment that I was in Two Section, Twenty-Five Platoon, Alamein Company. Just after this I was taken away from my mom and dad and still remember the instructor saying to them -

"It's ok, we are mom and dad now".

I was absolutely scared, I looked at my parents so I thought for the last time as I was led away to be issued the first bit of military kit I would ever receive. I was presented with a bright red tracksuit and a pair of the infamous Hi Tec Silver Shadow trainers, the elite training shoe of the British Army.

I was really upset as I did not get to say goodbye to my parents, I had a sick feeling inside, I was crying internally and wanting to run away. It felt to me like a prison sentence. Unknown to me the parents had been told to wait for us in the gym, so that we could say our final goodbyes before starting our training to become soldiers.

Mom was in bits, crying hard, and my dad was his normal stoic self, although I know now that he was hurting. We hugged it out and then I walked off to join my new family, I will never forget the last words that my dad said to me before I left.

"Son if you don't like it or cannot cope, you call us, and we will come straight back and pick you up".

This is what I needed to hear, as I knew that I could not let that happen and no matter how hard it was, I just did not want to let them both down!

A week went bye in a flash, I loved the routine, the hard-physical training and the discipline, come night-time though, if we ever did get anytime to ourselves, I would lie back and really miss home. I spent many a night as others did, crying into my pillow but trying to be quiet so as not to let anyone else hear me and think that I was weak. I was so nervous that I did not go for a number two all this time but eventually this passed. In fact, it passed with a bang and blocked the bog! I soon got into the swing of things.

We got beasted for the first 6 weeks and we were losing lads by the day. Some boys just could not handle it and had to quit. I often wonder what they do now. I had a great section commander called Corporal Reilly who was from Enniskillen Ireland, he was in the Royal Tank Regiment. Corporal Reilly was really clued up and had constructive advice for us. Do not get me wrong, he hated us but always pointed us in the right direction.

In my section we had some characters but a few to mention. There was Owen from Yorkshire and he even walked thick!! How he passed the entry I do not know! There was also Tyler Christopher from Birmingham, who reminded me of Howard from the Halifax advert. We are still great friends now and not to forget Ewan Stirling, who actually was from Stirling (Scotland). We were a close group and after doing everything together for the last six weeks, we did become family and without these guys I would have struggled.

One stand-out moment that would change millions of lives forever, and one which I will never forget, and you or your families reading this will never forget, from my time at Harrogate, is what happened on the 11th September 2001. We had just finished on a range day at Strensall, Yorkshire and were boarding the coaches to head back to the AFC. On the bus the TVs were on. Everyone stood there watching footage of planes crashing into buildings. What were we watching? A film? The latest Hollywood blockbuster? if only! It was a horrific act of Terrorism. Four US aeroplanes are hijacked and flown deliberately into targets in the US. 3,000 people are killed. The attack is quickly blamed on al-Qaeda and its leader Osama Bin Laden who was then resident in Afghanistan. The World Trade Centre was no more. I remember feeling so angry and sickened that someone could do this to innocent people. This event would change history forever and it would certainly change my life along with everyone on that bus with me.

Corporal Reilly said "fellas, you know what this means?"

We did not have a clue,

"you trained at the right time, because you will be going to war now!"

Wow! Is this really happening? As a young lad a rush of excitement overcame me, I get to go and kill the baddies! I would get that chance - but not yet.

During our training at Harrogate, we completed everything you can imagine from learning to shave, how to iron our kit as well as how to survive in the field, how to fight, use and maintain weapon systems. I was loving it and I was quite good at it. All you needed to do was listen and do as you're told for the first six weeks. Simples!

I did not leave school with any GCSEs, but I did get NVQs in IT, Maths and English at Harrogate and as we were forced to do it, I excelled. I had the best of both worlds. At the time it did not occur to me, but those NVQs would later enable me to get a job as a Paramedic. I am so grateful of that opportunity now.

So, my next bit of advice: "if a window of opportunity appears, don't pull down the shade". (Tom Peters)

Rugby again, here we go, rugby, rugby, rugby! but here is why. I loved this sport, and I could not get enough of it. So, when the chance came for me to play at the AFC I jumped at the opportunity. We were training three times a week in between all our military sessions, this was heaven. I met some fantastic lads. The coaches, although still our instructors, were our teammates and it was as relaxed an atmosphere as it would be back home at my local club.

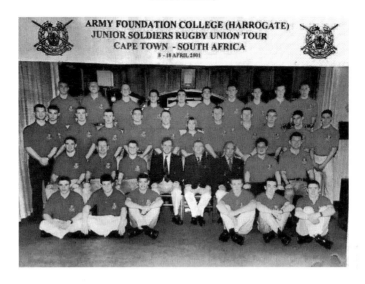

(Team photo before we set off to South Africa)

Another fantastic opportunity for me to represent the AFC and British Army came on a trip to South Africa. I could not believe it when I was selected. We got our Red Army t-shirts and were made to wear chinos, I'd never heard of them before, and were ready to jump on a plane to Johannesburg for our first stop, then on to Cape Town where we would play our games.

The tour was made up of lots of different characters from all social classes, however Rugby brought us together as a family. Some of the guys had never left their hometowns before and by joining the military and playing a sport they had this fantastic opportunity.

As members of our team went, we had Holden from St Helens. He was a fat lad and a woolly back or plastic scouse! We also had Campbell from Wick, which, if you look on a map of Britain, it's pretty much the highest point you can get in Scotland. He was a hard player, who was obviously left outside in the Scottish elements at birth. He was stone-faced and rugged, and I for one was glad he was on my side. We also had a lad called Wilson or (Dicky Grey) who he is now known, from Geordie land in the North East, who was to go on to serve with me in my final

Regiment.

Some other personalities with us on the trip from the DS (directing staff) were our main coaches, Sgt Douglas, and Sgt "TC" Roberts who years later, would be sadly killed in Iraq during war fighting operations. The sad reality was that another soldier accidently killed him. He was the first soldier to be killed in the 2003 conflict. I always remember him being such a constructive coach who would always get the best out of you, and I have tried to adopt this approach when coaching myself. It was a real honour to get to know him in the short time I had with him.

Another member of the coaching staff was Alfie Smith, he was our Physical Training Instructor (PTI) and someone we all feared, but respected as we knew his background.

Alfie Smith, whilst serving in the military in Northern Ireland, was convicted of murder for an incident he was involved in whilst manning a vehicle check point (VCP) in Northern Ireland. A car sped through a checkpoint where he and other soldiers were working. A volley of rounds or (bullets if your non-military) were fired. Smith fired four of them and it was said that the last one of those four hit and killed the passenger in the car. He was sentenced to life imprisonment which was later overturned.

As young wannabe soldiers we looked at this man as a God-like figure. He was not only an infantry soldier, but he had actually killed someone for real. For us, he had an aura around him - that same one that the career office sergeant did when I joined. Naively I wanted to be a soldier to kill the baddies! That's how childish I still was at 16, but still had 6 more years before I would have to make that call to kill or not.

Before our first game against Charleston Hill Senior Secondary School, (I know long winded name sorry), we were staying in a place called Stellenbosch. For those who do not know, its wine territory. Obviously, we were all under eighteen and never done wine tasting before, so we thought it be a great idea to give it a go. A decision we would later regret. Bearing in mind we had to play in the evening, half of the team took the plunge and sampled some local produce. It was fucking awful, however little did we know that to do the wine sampling correctly we had to look, smell, taste and spit. This as you can imagine never happened and we all got absolutely smashed.

Three hours before kick-off, Alfie Smith was beasting us all to within an inch of our puny lives. We were throwing up everywhere and we were punished severely. Not holding any grudges, they soon whipped us back into shape to face a very well-organised side and we were narrowly beaten. It was a good game of rugby-playing against kids from a privileged background. Following this match, we had two other games lined up.

We next played Trafalgar High School. This school was the first school in Cape Town for students of colour. The school also took a leading role in protesting against the Apartheid policies. Students at this school clearly came from very tough backgrounds and to look at them as we did, they had no one of size to intimidate us, so stupidly we thought it was going to be an easy day at the office.

How wrong was I? We were kicked, punched and eye-gouged from the first minute to the eightieth. I had never experienced anything like it in my life, it was a full-on battle of attrition, they may not have been big kids but bloody hell, they could rush in and get some digs in!

It took us a while to gain some control, we had to do this by a pack method. Two big lads would have to pin one of their players down, and I and others would have to punch them whilst they were pinned, it was the only way we could do it! I was 16 and, granted, I didn't have the biggest punch on me but when I gave it my all to give them a dig to the jaw, they would just smile! They were unbelievable kids who had obviously been brought up with tough love. What an experience!

We won the game on the scoreboard, but I am not sure about on the field. We shook hands and as of the end of any game of rugby, there were absolutely no hard feelings at all -great people they really were.

The final game of the tour is one I would never forget. We were privileged enough to play against Langa Township. Langa Township is 3 kilometres by 3 kilometres and is a suburb where during the Apartheid, black people were sent to live. Around seventy thousand people live in this small space. There poverty and unemployment are rife, and, sadly for the inhabitants, opportunity is limited. To be given this opportunity to see how these people live was a humbling one. This township at the time made up for fifty-five percent of the murders in Cape Town. It was a very lawless neighbourhood, so when it came to be playing them at rugby, we were all quite concerned about how the game would play out.

The pitch did not have a blade of grass on it and it was as dry as the desert. The players who we would face were on the other side of the pitch and were playing bare foot! We thought that surely, we wouldn't be playing them without boots on! We were! They played with different coloured strips on, no boots and as before they wanted a scrap. There was not much rugby played at all but this time we won the on-field battle and we also managed a draw on the scoreboard. These kids clearly had nothing, and it was a highlight of my trip until....

"They stole the fuckin' bus with all our kit and equipment on, the bastards!!!!"

Following this, we were able to visit Robin Island where Nelson Mandela was imprisoned. I even managed to see his cell and afterwards, I would never moan about military accommodation again. His cell was tiny, and he clearly would have had a horrendous time there. Another highlight was getting to climb Table Mountain in Cape Town. It is a beautiful mountain with such amazing views. We were all very privileged to be part of this trip.

Following a fantastic year at AFC Harrogate we were trained soldiers or so I thought. I had gained NVQs, I knew how to use weapon systems, I could look after myself in the field and also, I could administer first aid to my fellow soldiers, what a feeling this was. I got to show off in front of my family and friends with the added extra of being awarded "Best RA Soldier". Best RA (Royal Artillery) recruit was a massive achievement for me. Out of hundreds of recruits I got this award. I was absolutely buzzing and to that date the proudest of my life, I had achieved something meaningful.

Before our passing-out parade we had to choose what Regiment we wanted to serve with. As I said earlier, I had always wanted to be a "Para" like the recruitment sergeant at the Careers Office and like Lee Clegg, a stone-faced killer. However, I was head hunted by one of the most professional soldiers I would ever know: Bombardier Steve Newton or "Stevienewtron" as he was known. He was robotic like the Terminator and as fit as a greyhound. He was also as switched-on as can possibly be. He persuaded me rather than joining The Parachute Regiment, which is an infantry unit, to join his Regiment instead which was the 7TH Parachute Regiment Royal Horse Artillery. Yes, I know what you are thinking! How do you get horses to parachute from planes? My mind was made up when he told me that not only do we wear the "maroon machine" (Beret) and jump out of planes, we have the best rugby team in the British Army. I was easily bought when it came to rugby.

CHAPTER 4

<u>The Regiment</u>

7 Para RHA is the primary artillery supporting unit for airborne forces of 16 Air Assault Brigade.

The unit came into existence as 7th Parachute Light Regiment Royal Horse Artillery, following the re designation of 33rd Parachute Light Regiment Royal Artillery (also known as 33rd Parachute Field Regiment RA) on 27 June 1961. It can however trace its airborne heritage back to the 53rd Air landing Light Regiment, RA.

The designation was marked by the changing of beret badges from the 'Gun' to the 'Cypher', the changing of pennants and a march past led by the commanding officer, Lt Col Caulfield MBE. The salute was taken by Brigadier Northern MBE who also read out the following message from the Director Royal Artillery, Maj Gen Bate:

"Until today the Royal Horse Artillery has been confined to the support of Cavalry and Armour, a role which demands exceptional ability, quickness of thought and action. It is for this reason that the Royal Horse Artillery has been, ever since Napoleonic times, a Corps d'elite.

Under modern conditions the parachute role demands qualities in its officers and other ranks even more exacting than that required of the Royal Horse Artillery in its traditional role; for this reason its officers and other ranks have always been volunteers and specially selected. This Regiment has already established a proud and splendid tradition. As part of the spearhead of the strategic reserve it is very right and proper that it should now become part of the Royal Horse Artillery.

I know that this change of status is welcomed by the whole Regiment of Artillery. In sending you my best wishes or your success in both peace and in battle I believe I cannot do better than to voice the views of Her Majesty, Our Captain General; she has said that the change now to take place is 'entirely in keeping with the traditions that have made the Royal Horse Artillery famous.' "

In the same year 7 Para Lt Regt RHA was re-equipped with the Italian designed 105mm Pack Howitzer L5 and employed alongside the 4.2-inch mortar. The unit was renamed as 7th Parachute Regiment RHA in 1966.

Over the years, 7 PARA RHA have supported operations of 16 Parachute Brigade in the Near East, Aden and Radfan, Northern Ireland, as well as UN operations in Cyprus.

The Regiment was re-appointed as 7th Field Regiment RHA in 1977, after the 1975 Defence Review, but returned to the Airborne fold in 1983, once more designated 7th Parachute Regiment RHA for the new 5th Airborne Brigade. Further Battery operations to Northern Ireland followed in the 1980s and early 1990s, along with another deployment on the UN mission to Cyprus in 1994.

Batteries of 7 PARA RHA also took part in operations in Bosnia, and later Kosovo in the troubled Balkan region in the mid to late 1990s, helping to ensure 7 PARA RHA was retained as an integral part of 16 Air Assault Brigade, following the army reorganisations in 1999.

In the new millennium, operations of 16 Air Assault Brigade have seen 7 PARA RHA supply crucial fire support for operations in Macedonia, Afghanistan (Fingal) Iraq (Telic) and more recently, the deployments to Afghanistan as part of the ongoing Herrick operations.

Before I got to my regiment, I needed to complete phase two

training. I was to move from my home in Penny Pot Lane AFC Harrogate to Larkhill in Salisbury. This is where I was to complete my trade training to join the regiment. I would be trained on the L118 105MM light gun. The L118 Light Gun is a 105-millimetre towed howitzer. It was originally produced for the British Army in the 1970s has been widely exported since. It has a maximum firing range of 17.2 kilometres and a rate of fire of 6 to 8 rounds per minute. The 105MM light gun as it says in the title can be towed across rough terrain but can also be lifted by helicopter with crew on board, and deployed by parachute, which makes it a very versatile weapon system.

Over the next few weeks we were to learn everything about this piece of equipment. This would include how to fire the weapon, clean the weapon and how to maintain its readiness to fire. As I said before this was boys with toys! I love getting dirty and I love grafting. Picking up heavy pieces of equipment, loading artillery shells into the breach and firing it was the ultimate experience knowing that someone on the other end of it was getting the good news.

The aim of this equipment was to support the infantry on the ground. We could be as far away as 17.2 kilometres from the infantry and still manage to drop a single round of artillery accurately on the enemy. We were affectionately known as drop shorts or long-range snipers. One of the ammunition types we could use with this gun was the L 31 high explosive, 105-millimetre shell which comprised of high tensile steel body filled with RDX /TNT, fitted with the user select fuse. The user select fuse was essential in choosing whether the shell would explode on impact called point detonating or could be set for airburst to inflict more damage on the enemy in the open.

(brothers in arms, members of 7 PARA RHA in a charity rugby match for Pilgrim Bandits)

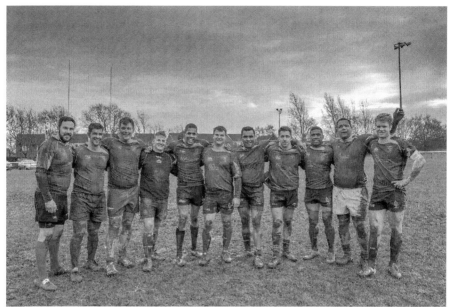

This type of ammunition had a lethal splinter distance of 40 metres. If you were anywhere in that radius you would be like a pineapple and blown to chunks. Not only could we deliver in - direct fire on the enemy in high explosive form, we could supply smoke and illumination at night to aid our infantry colleagues on the ground. A little later in the story, you will find out how the light gun was used during battles in Iraq and Afghanistan.

So, I passed my level 2-gun course with no problems at all I was then ready to move on to my next phase of training which was my car driving test. I could not believe my luck when they told me that we were eligible to get my full driving licence all paid for by the Army. Not only being in the Military, so far give me education in the form of NVQs, a trip to South Africa playing rugby, a trade as a level 2 gunner, but now they're going to teach me to drive and gain my full licence.

I was living the dream right now for sure! I met my instructor on the first day and I jumped into a blue Vauxhall Corsa to start my lessons. It is a good job I was already prepared for this as when I was a young boy around 13 or 14, I used to take my dad's old brown knackered Capri off the drive for a spin. One morning

I pulled off the drive with Diane, my parent's neighbour of many years shouting!

"Get back here now David before I call the police! You're too young to drive that and you could kill someone"!

Laughing, as I pulled off up the street to the top of Littlewood Lane, I chucked a right turn down to the Coal Truck Island and back again. This time is a little bit different as the Army were funding this for me, and I had to be professional and make sure I passed it because if I didn't, I'd face the wrath of being back squadded, and not being able to go to my regiment in a timely manner would not look good at all.

Passed my test with two minor faults - happy days! It was now time to take some leave and get ready to join my regiment. This would prove to be a very frightening experience to begin with.

CHAPTER 5

Reporting for Duty

I enjoyed my leave! I drank loads of beer, played the little bit of rugby and enjoyed showing off to all my friends. I was being an all-round knob if I am honest. At this point I'd passed phase one training to become a soldier, I had passed phase two training to get a trade under my belt, I could also now drive, which many of my friends from back home could not do. I believe I turned into an over-confident arrogant prick thinking I was better than everyone else. Boy, was I in for a massive surprise?

I reported for duty in my new home which would be Lille barracks, Aldershot in Hampshire. Aldershot had been home of the British army forever, but more Importantly for me it had been the home of the Airborne Forces for 50 years. It was an infamous place, known for all the pubs which all the different Airborne units frequented. I was a brand-new airborne gunner, and pretty much fresh meat on the table. I soon regretted being a prick back home and now it was time for me to step up into the big boys' world and try and become a Paratrooper myself.

I remember my first day walking up to the guard room absolutely shitting myself. I made sure I was well presented and turned out, I entered the guard room and there were about 3 or 4 paratroopers behind the desk just glaring at me. As I walked through the doors to the guard room, I made sure I dropped all of my kit to the left by some chairs in a nice neat pile and then prepared to march up to the desk and report for duty. Before I could even do this, I was met with

"Don't just leave your shit there you fuckin hat! "grunted one of the Paratroopers.

When I looked back, I was so scared reporting to the Careers Office for my interview, this time was that experience was on steroids, I could have cried. I was all alone with no other recruits to take the pressure off me. I gathered my composure, marched up to the desk instead.

"Gunner Bentley reporting for duty staff!"

I was met with the reply," I don't give a fuck who you are! What are you marching for you lunatic? Pick up all your shit, go to the I battery gun sheds, see the Staff Sergeant and he will sort you out, now get out of my sight you fucking lizard!"

This was the warmest welcome I ever had; I must admit. The Lance Bombardier in question who directed this abuse at me would in years to come be a good friend of mine. He is also now member of the Special Boat Service (SBS) So like in Harry Potter, he cannot be named.

Luckily for me, at the time I arrived at Lille Barracks, Aldershot, the rest of the regiment were on exercise in Salisbury, so the abuse I sustained was just minimal. I got squared away by the staff Sergeant, picked up some extra kit and was given directions to my room. I was told by the Staff Sergeant that I was to be in I Parachute Battery, Bulls troop. I knew there are different Batteries in the regiment, but I thought to myself that I really need to start cluing myself up on the Regiment. Soon I will meet the rest of the lads and if I don't know anything about it, I was going to get some shit and maybe even some beatings.

Let me give you a history lesson on I parachute battery, Bulls Troop. The Battery was formed on the 1st of February 1805 as I troop Horse Artillery at Colchester, Essex as I Horse Artillery Battery of the British Army. Captain Robert Bull was appointed to command and he took it to the Iberian Peninsula in August

1809, where it served until 1814. It arrived too late for the Battle of Talavera, but thereafter took part in most of Wellington's major actions of the Peninsula War, including Bussaco (1810), Fuentes De Onoro (1811), Ciudad Rodrigo, Badajoz, Salamanca, and Bergus (1812), Vitoria, San Sebastian, The Bidassoa and the Nive (1813) and Bayonne (1814).

The Battery and the Regiment have been involved in every major conflict since 1805, which include the Napoleonic wars, The First and Second World Wars, Operation Telic in Iraq, Operation Herrick in Afghanistan along with other peace support missions in the Balkans and Northern Ireland.

Our most important anniversary of the year is, Driver's Day which is on the 5th of May every year, which celebrates the action at Fuentes De Onoro during the Peninsula war.

Being the new guy at the regiment, I was known as either NIG (Newly Enlisted Gunner), Crowbag or Crap Hat. I was not allowed to speak to anyone and only speak when spoken to. The difference between me to the rest of the guys was that I had not passed the selection course that all Paratroopers must pass. To serve in The Airborne Forces, I would need to pass the infamous Pegasus Company, or P Company as its more commonly known.

Over the next few weeks and months, I really kept my head down, worked hard and just did as I was told. We had battery PT every day at 7:00am and I would make sure I was up and ready to go, to prove that I could mix with these airborne Gods. I was doing everything I could to be the grey man, not cause any trouble, and when asked to do something, I made sure I did it to the best of my ability every time.

I joined the regiment to play rugby, and secondly become a Paratrooper and jump out of planes. However, because I had not passed P Company or even had chance to try it yet, this made me ineligible to do anything inside the regiment apart from the really shit jobs. I remember one night lying in my bed and a Senior bloke come through the door, pissed as a fart, and told me to "get down the shop and get me some fags you hat!"

He was a big, stocky chap and I did not want to annoy him, but I seemed to have stepped over the line when I asked him for the money.

"Money!?" he said, "Use your own fucking money!"

Let me get this right, I had to get out of my pit, get dressed, walk 3 miles to the shop just to get some cigarettes, out of my own money. This was clearly not the life I wanted at the moment. I was trying my best to get on and not cause any issues, but because I had not earned my maroon beret and yet to pass P Company, I remained a target of abuse until I had done so. I needed the opportunity to pass this course sooner rather than later, I just thought the abuse was the norm however now looking in it was direct abuse and bullying, but I did not know any different.

The worst time for me in the regiment in the early days was mealtimes. If you were not parachute trained, you were made to eat last and sit behind all the other para trained soldiers with a barricade in between us so they did not have to look at us. We were made to feel the lowest of the low. Sometimes it got that bad, I would not go and eat, I was that worried. Thankfully, this does not happen anymore, and I would not wish this treatment on anyone, it was just the norm. No encouragement was given to me whatsoever and anything I wanted to do I had to go out and do it myself. Do not get me wrong, the battery fitness was harder than anything I had done before, whether that was on my own in Civvy Street or during training at the Army Foundation College.

After a few months I got the opportunity I was waiting for, a place on Pre Para. Pre Para is six weeks build-up phase or so they sell it as, a punishing beat up to make sure we are ready to be selected to go up to Catterick to have a crack at P company.

By the time I was ready to start Pre Para there were other boys who had now joined the unit, and I was so glad, this meant that at last I did not have all the abuse and shit coming my way constantly. It was the other lads turn to get some.

This was the time where I met one of my best friends, Sean Dunbabbin, aka Babs or Rat Boy. To this day Babs any myself remain great friends, or even go as far to say brothers. I would not know it at the time, but Babs and I would be peas in a pod, doing everything together for the next few years. Babs. How would I describe him? If you have ever seen the film Beetlejuice, and you recall the waiting room scene, there is a monster in the room with the smallest head you have ever seen, looking like a raison on top of two shoulders, this was Babs. He was a skinny lad from Bolton, complete with ginger hair, although he reckons it's Afghanistan Sunset. This bloke was as fit as ten men and just like a little terrier that you could fit in your pocket and break out in case of emergency. He is a real legend.

It was great to have a friend in Babs when starting Pre Para as I knew it was going to be nails, and although looking forward to the challenge, I was nervous at the prospect of failure. We cracked on with Pre Para and we were under two Physical Training Instructors (PTIs). Andy and Dave (were the PTIs) and Zak was Dave's dog who was a chocolate Labrador. Andy and Dave were, and still are, machines of the highest order, and it was their job to push us to our limits and make sure that at the end we were ready to go (up the road) to Catterick to complete the infamous P Company.

Failure rates for Pre Para were high, and even more so when it came to P Coy. We would typically do two or three events each day over the Aldershot training area, where P Coy used to be held. Each day would consist of quick runs, loaded marches and gym sessions. Sounds constructive? It was Hell on Earth! I never thought I would make it to the end of the day in some cases, let alone finish the course. I was a fit, young lad at the time but even so, I had never pushed my body as hard as this. I soon realised that it was not all about physical strength, but more so mental toughness to crack on when it becomes hard. Over the next few weeks, we got ragged physically and mentally, my feet were in shit state, back scarred from carrying my bergen. Sadly, some lads fell by the wayside, some picked up injury and some purely did not want it enough and had a sudden realisation that this was not for them.

I pushed myself as hard as I could, and I was really starting to feel it. The constant body aching, tiredness and mental fatigue and pressure put on by the staff, constantly seeing if we had the minerals to become Airborne Soldiers. Babs however, was a little twat, he breezed through it all without a sweat, but to his credit helped others including me along the way.

Every morning we would have spot checks on our kit and if, for example, our black water bottles were not full to the brim, you would be wearing it. Emphasis was put on fitness, determination, supporting others and kit and equipment.

The weeks went quickly and from about twenty-five blokes who started Pre Para there were only around twelve left. Myself and my mate Babs were in the twelve, along with Ryan and Jacko with whom we gelled on the course.

It was the last day of Pre Para and those of us who were left were told to get on parade, to see if we had done enough to earn the right to head up the road to attempt P Coy.

I was feeling tense, nervous "Had I done enough?" "Does my face fit?" all the doubts entered my head, sickening feeling that if I had not done enough, I would have to go through all that blood, sweat and tears again.

"Dunbabbin!" shouted the staff.

"Sir" Babs replied.

"Pass!"

I was chuffed for him, but there was never any doubt, it was a stroll in the park for him. Jacko and Ryan had the same result and they were through, my turn next.

It was a pass! and seven of us out the twelve remaining were off to attempt Pre-Parachute Selection, P COY at Catterick. I was made up but, felt physically and emotionally drained. Imagine how the guys felt who went through all that pain, to get to the end and be told that they were not ready? Some of those people have given everything. Later, you will find out why only the best and most suitable pass this course and no quota was given, you either meet the standards or not, simple as that.

Only a couple of days to recover and then we were heading north.

CHAPTER 6

Pegasus Company

P re-Parachute Selection must be undertaken by all British Army Candidates who wish to be considered for Parachute Training and who have not already undergone a strenuous form of training such as UK special Forces.

The aim of P Coy is to test physical fitness, determination, and mental robustness under conditions of stress, to determine whether and individual has the self-discipline and motivation required to serve with Airborne Forces.

Training at P Coy culminates in a series of eight tests undertaken over a five-day period. All Arms candidates, such as I, would have a further two and a half weeks Pre Para screening before we could attempt P Coy itself or Test Week as it is known.

We all turned up to Catterick on the Sunday before P COY, got into our accommodation and got our heads down for the night ready for our first day. Screening day, following successful Pre Para with our own units, we needed to pass the screening day, if we didn't it would be a very lonely trip back down to Aldershot, not only to get ridiculed by everyone but it would mean that we would have to start all over again.

The tests on the first day consisted of a Combat Fitness Test or CFT, which is an eight mile squadded march, carrying a 35lb bergan (plus water) and weapon system, to be completed in 1 hour 50 mins or less.

The Trainasium test, which is an Arial confidence course and following this, a basic fitness assessment which comprised of a 1.5 mile run preceded by a 1.5 mile warm up to be completed in a time of 9 mins 30 seconds or less.

This was bloody day one and if we failed any part of this screening, we were gone, returned to unit (RTU).

Off we went! Whilst on P Coy you are being assessed from the minute you arrive until the minute you go, looking at your posture, interaction levels and attitude. Everything had to be spot on, but this day was all about the pass, the rest could wait until tomorrow.

Squadded march was not a problem as we had done these previously to the time, so we were confident that we could crack it here, with our boots slightly undone at the top as we all had shins that felt like they were on fire, while trying to keep in step with the man in front. We Tabbed (tactical advance to battle) most of the way, but now and then would be met by the cries of "Prepare to double" "double march" and we would leg it in an attempt to keep up. We sailed in under the time and thought to ourselves "yes we have a rest now the trainasium"

The Trainasium, if you were stood next to it, does not look much other than a high pile of scaffolding that you would see around buildings etc, however it has proven over the years to break people due to their fear of heights. It had many features but today was just a simple confidence check to see if we could progress to day 2.

We had to climb a set of ladders up to the top of the Trainasium which stood at a height of 17 metres or 55ft, it does not sound much but without safety equipment it did put a few off.

We had to climb as high as we could and stand on 2 parallel bars. There was nothing but fresh air below us and we were given a few commands and had to react straight away too, or we failed. I stood up straight and was told to shuffle along the bars! So after taking a deep breath, with my head up I did and shuffled away until I was told to stand still. I was then met by 2 knuckles on the bars so I would not be able to shuffle any further. My next command was to touch my toes! So, I did no problem, there was a little bit of wind which was not from my arse, although it could easily have been! I was then told to step over the knuckles! Been 55ft up in the air, stood on 2 bars, without any safety equipment I felt quite uneasy, however I composed myself, put the weight on my left leg and lifted my right foot over the lump and then did the same again for my left, I had done it!

"Right stop showing off! get down".

I did. That was now 2 tasks out of 2 completed. The last test was to come.

3 miles to go now, a 1.5 mile warm up, which was bollocks, it was in fact a beasting for 1.5 miles, then we had to complete the other 1.5 miles in under 9 minutes and 30 seconds. My heart was pounding out my chest, white saliva running down my face and I had a wheeze in my throat. I felt like I was going to die! However, I wanted it that badly that I gave it everything and came in just in the time! I was relieved and as I was just catching my breath when an instructor stood behind us, directing a few other guys also behind us to one side, they obviously had not made the time and that was them done! Gone! RTU'd!

Day 1, and screening was now complete. I am now on P Coy and the worst is yet to come. I was now the proud owner of a P Coy number, 41 that is me! From now I will not be referred to as anything else. Over the next 2 and a half weeks we would be on the build-up phase for test week. Bearing in mind, I had already just completed 3 weeks of beat-up to get ready for this point. Everyone was in the same boat and clearly falling to bits.

We did not know at the time, but over the next few weeks we would cover around 94 miles in various forms, it was to be physically and mentally tough however with some constructive elements.

We would be having 2 or 3 sessions a day which would include loaded marches, hill reps and gym sessions which all aimed to fatigue us for test week and to see what we were made of. Along with the arduous physical sessions we would also have lessons on First Aid, map reading and field craft all whilst under intense pressure and monitoring. We completed night navexs in teams and learnt how to fight with bayonets, this day still stands out in my mind.

The day we completed bayonet training was the most exhausting I can remember, the reason for this was that the staff would get us so fired up before we learnt how to use our bayonets that we actually felt like we were going to war.

How did they do this? Well as normal they got us into our sections and beasted us physically with press-ups, stress positions and just generally fucking us around. We were tired and fed up already however, they took us to a field in which we could see targets set up and waiting for us. There was a calmness suddenly. A corporal said in a soft voice,

"Right gents, today you are going to learn how to............" All the sudden his voice changed, and he continued ....

"Kill the fucking enemy, with airborne aggression and a bayonet".

I was ready and felt like I did when I was having a fight back at school. They stirred us up by saying things about our families, calling us weak and pathetic! I could not write the exact words, but you get the idea. I had never received so much abuse, but there was a reason for it. After a few hours of this mental torture they give us instruction on the technical aspects of bayonet fighting and use of the Hight Port (holding your rifle and bayonet across your chest in a controlled manner. The other was the En-Garde! position which was ready to attack.

We were pumped and I admit lost an element of control but this was part of the plan, we were forced to shout "kill, attack, kill , attack " and adopt the high port position and then the En - Garde.

The corporal was shouting,

"what makes the grass grow?",

"blood! blood! blood!" We replied!

They were purposely holding us back and building the hate inside of us, I wanted to kill, and it didn't matter what! Psychologically, we were subjected to so much information that instinctively we had to process the one thing and that was to thrust a bayonet into a target, through the centre of the chest and keep going until the target was dead. You may think I don't have it in me, or I would or could never do that to another human being but I learnt then, and down the line, that if you need to do it under that much mental pressure you will, that is fact.

It was my go, the staff were in my face and I had tears rolling down my cheeks, cam cream in my eyes from the sweat off my head, I was not crying but I was so fired up I could of taken on a whole Army myself. Call it brain washing or whatever, but to be a paratrooper I had to have this edge and a switch to go from killer one minute and switch on to be a thinking soldier the next. This is what the drill was about.

"En garde! I shouted.

I walked towards my target, screaming as loud as I could, using every bit of anger and power I could muster. With an almighty roar, I thrusted my bayonet into the target and fucking destroyed it! Let us just say that if you saw it going on in the street, you would be highly disturbed by our actions.

Yes, fair enough it was a dead pig, but blood, texture and smell are all the same and in the frame of mind I was in, it would not of mattered what it was, we were all killers this day.

Following this training we were all left alone. I found out later that as we were subjected to this torture it was highly likely that later on, there could have been a murder investigation, as the lads were on the edge of breaking and it took some time for things to calm down.

Later, in the story you will see how elements of this helped me and my mates out in a real-life scenario.

CHAPTER 7

Test Week

Babs, Ryan (who was known as Teeth), and myself had all done enough to reach Test Week or P Company. It was a culmination of our beat-up training and the part that was pass/fail.

The Tests: we had to pass in the final week to earn the coveted maroon beret.

10 Mile March (Wednesday morning) The 10-mile march is conducted as a squad, over undulating terrain with each candidate carrying a bergen (backpack) weighing 35 lbs (plus water) and a weapon. The march must be completed in 1 hour and 50 minutes. TA candidates have 2 hours. I found this event tough; it was squadded and trying to keep the gaps closed always was hard going, especially if you had a short arse in front of you as I did. The timings to complete this test are tight and you must run much of the way, a real shin burner. I found myself getting slowly pushed out of the pack in the last couple of miles, and I could see the squad up ahead of me. "Number 41 get your fucking arse up there!" was the small bit of encouragement I needed. I had never physically hurt so much in my life, but I managed to drive through the pain and finish strong with the rest of the lads. Number one test down.

Trainasium (Wednesday afternoon) The Trainasium is an aerial confidence course which is unique to P Coy. To assess the suitability for military parachuting, the Trainasium tests a candidate's ability to overcome fear and carry out simple activities and instructions at a height above ground level. The event is a straight pass or fail. This was the easiest test of them all, as very straightforward in what needed to be done. As I mentioned earlier, I did not mind the heights and the climbing was wholesome fun. As we did back on screening day we had to get to the top, touch our toes which was not a problem, then move on to two more exercises which were a little more interesting. The illusion jump, I was stood on a platform looking across at the other platform, thinking that there was no way I can jump across there from a standing position, it's too far! It was below the plank I was standing on; it gave the illusion of being further away than it was. Without time to think too much about it I had the command "standby GO!" Off I went and landed the jump with precision. My legs hit the plank before my mind had had chance to process the jump, this was to test the ability of a candidate to jump on command, rather than making the decision himself. The next test was the run jump run punch. We had to run along a plank jumping from one plank to the other until we met a final opening where we had to run as hard and as fast as we could, jump and at the same time punch so our arms would go through the cargo net at the end, and then we were to lock ourselves off. If you did not lock out, it was P Company over, as it was 25 ft of nothing to the ground, we had a few lads who had fractured their ankles.

Log Race (Thursday morning) A team event with 8 individuals carrying a 60kg log over 1.9 miles of undulating terrain. Without a doubt, the hardest event on P Coy. Our 8-man section were belly down waiting for the scmooley (Flare) to go up, signalling the start of the race. Off we went, and we all ran as fast as we could to our logs, basically, it was a telegraph pole. I was on the rear of the log with my left wrist attached to a rope. As soon as we picked up the log the pain hit me like nothing else, I had ever experienced in my life, it was awful. Pain was shooting up my arm, into my shoulder, along with excruciating pain in my lower back. The Lads and I were absolutely hanging out of our arses. We lost a couple of lads within the first 500 metres which did not make life easier for any of us who were left. We had to keep a straight arm with all the weight on it over undulating terrain to simulate taking ammunition to the front line of a battlefield. Aggression here was the key, I was sucking the air in from every hole, a nice white foam appeared around my gob and all I could think to shout was "come on, keep driving!" I had nothing else in my brain that I could process at this time. We heard a rumour that if you come off the log on P Coy you would fail the whole course; I was not about to let this happen. I think still to this day I have never felt anything like it, and when I have a tough day I just think of the log, get a grip of myself and say, it could be worse!

It was over the one that I had been most worried about, we completed the 1.9-mile route with 5 lads still left on the log which was a bonus. Other logs were not that fortunate, and the DS staff had to help some as they had 4 or 5 come off theirs. My wrist was bleeding, and I still bear the scars to this day, but I am proud that I completed it and did not let my mates down.

Steeplechase (Thursday afternoon) An individual test with candidates running against the clock over a 1.8-mile cross country course. The course features several 'water obstacles' and having completed the cross-country element, candidates must negotiate an assault course to complete the test. The march must be completed in 19 minutes or under to score 10 points; TA candidates have 20 minutes 30 seconds. We had not much time to recover from our thrashing on the log of death and had to prep for the Steeplechase. This was a cross country run like few others. We started on our belly again and a thunder flash set us off. It was an all-out sprint to the start of the course and that's when all-out war broke out. We got to a funnel at the start of the water obstacles and as blokes wanted to get to the finish first, the fighting commenced. I was punched, pushed, stood on and that is before I even got to an obstacle. However, I gave as good as I got, dropping a few with my elbow and dropping the nut on one bloke as he was trying to pull me back. I loved a scrap, so this was my kind of event. I was flying until the last bit of the assault course, where there was a bulky frame that we had to negotiate with a rope to slide down at the end. I got up over the frame no problem, until I slid down the rope, my hands lost grip and I whacked my bollocks on the knuckle at the end of the rope and then dropped to the deck like a naughty sailor. With my eyes streaming and my balls in my stomach, I had to get up fast and take control of my body to ensure I made the time. I did so, just!

2 Mile March (Friday morning) The 2-mile march is conducted over undulating terrain with everyone carrying a bergen (backpack) weighing 35lbs (plus water) and a weapon. A helmet and combat jacket are also worn. The march must be completed in 18 minutes or under. TA candidates have 19 minutes. With my balls just about recovered, we had to conquer the 2 miles. This we were used to doing and it was a straight-out sprint as fast as you can for 2 miles, just make sure you come in under 18 mins. We set off and I saw Babs zoom away like Sonic the Hedgehog, he must have finished in 15 mins, myself however 17 mins with plenty of time to spare! Happy days! We had the luxury of a weekend of rest and by heck did I need it! I was suffering with tendonitis, blisters and feeling so run down from all the events so far. What I should have done was sleep and eat, instead in true soldier fashion, we pissed it up all weekend.

Endurance March (Monday) A squadded march conducted over 20 miles of severe terrain. Everyone carries a bergen (backpack) weighing 35lbs (plus water and food) and a weapon. The march must be completed in under 4 and a half hours. TA candidates do not undertake this event. This was a long old slog over Warcop Ranges, my type of pace but we certainly felt it after completing the 20 miles. We did not have smart watches or phones back then, but I would have certainly liked to see the elevation gains from that day. Babs obviously found it quite easy as I caught him texting a bird during the event. If he got caught, we would have all been punished severely, and he would have gotten the kicking of his life.

Stretcher Race (Tuesday morning) Teams of 16 men carry a 175lbs stretcher over 5 miles. No more than 4 men carry the stretcher at any given time. Students wear webbing and carry a weapon. Another tough challenge this one. It seems easy that only 4 men out of 17 carry the stretcher at one time, however over 5 miles this becomes quite a test. You have a 175 lb stretcher banging off your shoulder, sapping your legs and energy for short sharp periods, then you have to change and keep up at the rear of the stretcher where you can get a little bit of rest. Trying to keep up was tough and it all comes down to pure aggression and determination as well the willingness to help your mates out. We lost a few more on this event, some of the lads had already come off the log, so it was guaranteed to be curtains for them.

Milling (Tuesday afternoon) The final event of Test Week is 60 seconds of 'controlled physical aggression' against an opponent of similar height and weight. This was an interesting one minute of my life that I will never forget. We paraded at the gym and were paired off based on size and weight, I was facing an officer of a similar build but vastly different background. It was fantastic for me to be able to batter an officer! Or so, I thought. We were forced to stare each other out for about 20 mins before the event, he was looking into my eyes and was giving it a real go to psyche me out, but it was not working. I was laughing at him thinking that I would destroy him. It was Babs's turn before mine, and as always it was skins v shirts. We all sat in a square made up of those benches we all used in PE at school, with our hands up to support the fighters if they fell. The idea of milling was to attack constantly without defending yourself for one minute, switch on and switch off, controlled aggression.

I was worried for Babs, who I knew had never had a fight in his life. However, when the OC shouted his name, he was like a man possessed. He was battering this poor bloke who did not even know what planet he was on. Babs's fists were being powered by a Duracell battery! Wow Babs, fair play mate! My turn was coming up and this officer was still at it, staring me out and waffling on in his posh accent how he was going to batter me. So, here is how it went in the words of my good mate Babs:

"Initially stepping up to mill, you seemed very calm and collected, smashing the officer up with direct blows to the head, left right left, but once the officer got one shot in on you, you turned into a man possessed and you saw red! Ignoring the whole concept of controlled punches, your left arm wrapped around the officer's neck in a vice like grip, your right hand upper cutting the poor guys face 3 or 4 times until the fight was stopped and the officer hit the deck."

I was so fired up and really wanted to damage this person, the whole idea of milling was the controlled aggression. I completely lost it. My section commander calmed me down and although I lost it a bit, he said that in a one way fight I would not have learned anything. As the battle changed and I received incoming, it was all about overcoming that and adding more pressure to win. Another massive lesson for me and one again in Afghanistan would help me survive. The officer and I shook hands, as with rugby all was forgotten but I will never forget his words to me following our battle.

"Bentley I would take you fucking anywhere with me".

This meant the world and I had obviously earnt his respect as he had mine, what a legend.

The worrying part for me was the controlled aggression aspect, which later in the story would be the undoing of all I had worked hard for, when I was arrested and was facing a prison sentence.

P Coy was over and we would shortly learn our fate............

During the last few weeks we lost a few lads along the way and without a doubt it had been the toughest thing I had ever faced, mentally and physically, I knew I had given it my all. Was I the fittest? no. The fastest? No. Was I there at the end? Most certainly yes, I dug in blind to make sure I was there to support my mates, I just hoped it was enough.

We all paraded with our crap hats on ready to get the news. In the traditional way the OC would call out the remaining number and simply say "pass" or "fail". I was number 41 and the wait was horrendous. There were people passing who I knew I was as good as, but also people failing that surprised me. Number 38 was called,

"Number 38!"

The bloke next to me replied "Sir!" and came to attention,

OC replied "fail!",

he replied "Sir".

Clearly disappointed he then had to fall out of the squad and march to the rear of the parade and turn his back away from the rest of us and was now known as a failure. He had given everything and got to the end of test week to be told he had failed which was gut wrenching.

It was my turn ....

"Number 41"

"Sir" I replied whilst coming to attention,

"Pass",

"sir" I replied and at this moment I could have cried. I had passed P Company, the hardest military selection in the British Isles, other than special forces! I was now part of something special which meant I can now complete my parachute training becoming part of a band of brothers in the Airborne Forces. This was the proudest moment for me and for the rest of my family. I had achieved something special and was awarded my Maroon Beret to wear with pride. I am on my way to becoming a Paratrooper.

My P Company personal qualities scored above average on determination, above average on mental robustness, average for fitness, average for stamina, average on team spirit. As a youth there were lots of areas to improve clearly but a pass is a pass, and those Parachute Regiment Staff would not let any shit through that was for sure.

"Pain, it may last a minute, or an hour, or a day, or a year, but eventually it will subside and something else will take its place. If I quit, however, it lasts forever." (Lance Armstrong).

CHAPTER 8

Red On!

"You are about to carry out a parachute decent. You are to jump when the green light is displayed. Failure to do so constitutes disobeying a direct order and disciplinary action will be taken against you. In the event of the green light failing to operate, the number 1 will be dispatched on order of the PJI. You are to follow in your stick order and carry out a parachute decent. Failure to do so constitutes disobeying a direct order and disciplinary action will be taken against you." (Green Light Warning Order)

With P Company passed, I returned to my regiment full of pride and no longer having to wear a crap hat but a penguin instead. You cannot believe it, I passed one of the most physically and mentally demanding courses and I still had a shit nickname – penguin - meaning, all flap and no fly. A couple of good things came out though. The blokes who ridiculed me on day one and who would not even have pissed on me if I were on fire came up to me, shook my hand tightly and said fuckin respect Benny, as I would now be known. This, although not right felt amazing. I had earnt their respect a little. Until I had Parachute Wings on my arm, though, they would not acknowledge me fully. Another bonus was I could now play rugby for my regiment. We had an amazing team who had won the Army Cup at that time for the last 3 years.

I mentioned before that rugby was my saviour and it's true. I got out of doing that many shit jobs at the Regiment due to me being in the team. It was fantastic, although short lived, in our unit it was a good feeling being a tracksuit soldier for a while. Short lived indeed. The Regiment was part of 16 Air Assault Brigade which meant that all units in the Brigade are specially trained and equipped to deploy by parachute, helicopter, and air landing. The core role of our brigade was to keep the role of Air Assault Task Force Battlegroup, always held at high readiness to deploy worldwide for a full spectrum of missions, from non-combatant evacuation operations to war fighting operations. Pretty cool hey?

Rumblings were coming through to us about Iraq. I had heard a little bit about this place and knew that my uncle had gone to war in 1990 but that was about it. As an 18-year-old lad, I felt I was ready to take on the world if called upon and was very much of the mindset, For Queen and Country and for the lads. Although I had to grow up quickly and had been in the Army since I was 16, I was still very naïve and surrounded by similar young lads who just wanted to fight, get amongst the ladies, and go to war. The regiment had not been involved in any major conflicts for a little while, so everyone was keen to do their bit. Before this though, it was my turn to head down to RAF Brize Norton, to complete my Basic Parachute Course in sunny Oxfordshire, I could not wait.

We turned up at No 1 Parachute Training School, thinking we were the muts nuts, we were the only Army lads around on a RAF base we were going to run riot. As before I was with my little friend Babs and a few other lads this time, all waiting to sample jumping from a perfectly serviceable aircraft, exciting times.

Our predecessors obviously left their mark on the air force base, as our accommodation was right at the back of the centre, pretty much on the edge of the runway, in buildings that I can only describe as dog kennels! We were not bothered in the slightest, this was a jolly compared to P Company and we made sure that we had an enjoyable time. We settled in and got into a routine, we paraded at the Parachute School to get our introductions done and to find out what our course would involve.

We were briefed on the course in a massive hanger, which held a mock-up aircraft, a tower, better known as the fan, and flight swings, which we would learn to love like a family member.

Before we even got near a real aircraft, we had to complete our ground training and this consisted of kit familiarisation, drills, and floor work, i.e. how to do a "Para Roll".

To qualify as a military Parachutist, we had to conduct 8 parachute descents, varying in height, equipment used, single and sim sticks, and one decent at night. We started ground training and we learnt all about the kit we would use which was the Irvin Low Level Parachute or LLP for short, and the Irvin LLRP which was our reserve chute. We were taught emergency drills in case we got hung up outside the plane, which may sound fun although I did not fancy personally. We were taught how to deal with that situation, the main point being that you do not pull your reserve chute, or they will find 2 different body parts in 2 different counties. We got in the flight swings to practise our immediate action drills on exiting the aircraft, these really killed your balls, not meant for comfort at all.

We covered Drop Zone Hazards (DZ) landing in water, crashing into buildings, they really thought of everything. In WW2 there were airborne miss drops all over the country, so I suppose they had learnt from the past. We had scenario after scenario in those bastard swings, which included "Rigging lines rear", "rigging lines front" "Rigging lines right" I'm thinking bloody hell - just how close are we going to be next to each other? Very close was the answer, as close as half a second between each man.

The bit I was most worried about was an air steal! this occurred when one parachute drifts over another, causing the parachute at the bottom to deflate, and both sets of parachutes race to the ground one after each other, re inflating once in clear airspace, however if you hit the ground first with a half inflated canopy, you're in big trouble.

We were there, we got our practise equipment on, and boarded the mock-up plane. We were broken down into sticks, port and starboard, today I still cannot remember if that is left or right.

We cracked the drills that we were taught, and we all did a funny dance to the door following each other out of the mock aircraft. We were laughing and joking and not really taking it that seriously. This would change in the morning when we were to do our first real jump out of a Hercules C130 transport plane or, Fat Albert as we used to call him.

Jump day arrived, but the weather was due to be pretty crappy in the morning, so we had another go at The Fan, which was a high platform with a zipline attached that was meant to simulate, jumping from a plane and also how it felt to land.

I jumped out as we were taught shouting:

"one thousand, two thousand, three thousand, check canopy".

 We were trained to do this every time; this would represent the time needed for our canopies to fully inflate. I was bouncing around on this bloody wire and banged out a textbook parachute roll at the bottom. Little did I know that this roll would have been the last one I performed ever, as real time, you are about to find out, it does not happen.

Kit on, combat 95 trousers and issued boots, parachute smock, parachute helmet and of course LLP and LLRP parachute and reserve. No other kit was needed for our first jump. At the start of this chapter, there was a Green Light Warning order which was read out to us before any parachute decent. Any bottling it at the parachute doors means that you are out the Airborne Forces. I had not gone through hell and back on P Company, to fail at this point was not an option.

We walked out to the aircraft with extremely nervous looks on the lads' faces as well as lots of career laughing as we used to call it. Basically, people making shit jokes and nervously laughing back at them. This was real, I had never done anything like this in my life, I used to be scared of the bin man for God's sake, how can I be lobbing out of a plane? Babs and I sat close together as normal along with one of our Fijian brothers, Phil Tagavaka-tini or Tags. He put us at ease. He was a very big man who spoke softly but did worry us slightly when he started to pray.

"God be with you boys" I recalled him saying.

I replied, "Cheers Tags, at least we are covered now".

We got to the back of this massive green aircraft and we could smell the jet A1 fuel. I started to feel sick but there was no going back. We sat down, back to back on some red fold-down seats. I could see a few sick bags, which turned my stomach even more. We removed our LLRPs from our chest and strapped in, waiting for the Parachute Jump Instructors (PJIs) to finish off their checks. The PJIs were RAF personnel who choose to do this for a living, crazy people but incredibly supportive and relaxed with us. I could see the propeller's start turning out of a small window opposite, and a loud buzzing followed as the engines started to turn over. There were worried faces everywhere now.

With the propellers at full speed, a little bump we were off and rolling and began our taxi to the runway. After a couple of minutes, we stopped. It was extremely dark inside the aircraft with only a little light coming in through those small circular windows. The engines roared even louder; we were at maximum revs for take-off. All the lads on my side leaned to the left and we stayed in this position as we sped off down the runway, my stomach churning as we got airborne. We levelled off and all of us could sit upright again, another groaning sound at the undercarriage was housed.

(Me and Tags about to make a parachute decent)

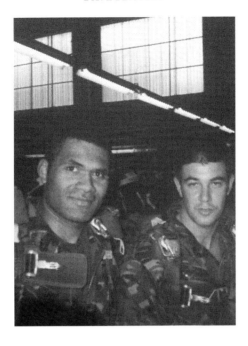

We knew it was only a short flight time from Brize Norton to the drop zone at Weston On the Green. We had had this brief already and were told to look out for the M40 motorway which ran right next to the DZ. This could be an awkward landing if we had to dodge traffic too! The time came to get prepared.

We got the command,

"stand up, fit equipment".

The drills we all hoped would kick in now. So, we stood, folded away the seats we were sat on, clipped our reserve chutes onto our hooks near our chest. Obviously now we were frantically checking them 50 times to make sure they were stuck on well. The PJIs then walked down the port and starboard sides of the aircraft pulling everyone's static line out the top of the main chute, hooking them on to a cable above our heads. We were good to go. As this was our very first jump, we would be at 1000ft in a single stick, that meaning only using one side of the aircraft on one pass at a time rather than both sides at the same time as normal. We had no equipment at all, that would make our lives a little easier this time.

Next command

"starboard stick, sound off for equipment check!"

This was the time that the first 6 of us would shout, whilst slapping each other on the back as hard as we could,

"6 ok, 5 ok, 4 ok, 3 ok, 2 ok,1 ok, starboard stick ok!".

This gave the PJI at the Parachute doors the nod that we were hooked up and ready to jump. I was number 3 in the door for my first jump and Babs was number 1, I was shitting myself so I had not a clue how he would feel stood right in the door, looking straight out, it must have been information overload for him. The PJI opened the Para door, a rush of air and light flooded into the aircraft. We could feel a big temperature change and we could also see all the fields, buildings, and cars below us. We were not that high, so everything was really moving quickly on the ground.

You could see the propellers spinning, that jet A1 smell now worse than before and nervous tension all around. We got the call "action stations!", on this command we all had to push up close as we can to each other, this was to enable the PJI to get us out the aircraft as quickly as possible in order for us to all land on the DZ instead of in water trees or the M40! The PJI signalled that the wind on the ground was 5 knots, he did this by blowing into his hand then holding his hand out like a high 5.

With tension building and never having been this nervous in my life, we got the p minus 2 min call. We were anxiously looking at the 2 lights above the para door, one red one green, remember the green light order, when that light is on we are off.

Now at stalling speed, Fat Albert was flying at around 120 mph. "Red ON" was the cry from PJI then we followed suit by shouting "Red ON!! This was it, no turning back. My stress levels were now through the roof and I am about to leap out of an aircraft side door! Without time to process, there was another scream of "Go!" The PJI was now counting "1, 2 and before I heard the next number which was me! I was out the door, following the men before me, I pushed myself out of the para doors as hard as I could, did I shout what I was supposed to? Did I bollocks?! The air took my breath away and all I recall is seeing the sky and the ground and feeling a tugging sensation behind my head. It felt like a lifetime but within seconds, I looked up and there was a canopy. Yes! I'm alive, get in! What a bloody relief, to be honest if there was not a canopy there, I dare say that I would probably be dead by now, as I was so scared and don't think my brain would have engaged for me to pull the reserve.

From all the noise of the aircraft there was now complete silence, you could have a conversation with the bloke next to you. I held on to my front 2 risers and drifted down towards the ground, which appeared to be coming at me quite quickly, however at least I was headed for grass and not the tarmac of a busy M40. There was a PJI on the ground with a loud hailer shouting "get tight", "feet together". The first 2 lads were down, their deflated canopies on the ground a couple of seconds before, I pulled down hard on my risers, got my feet together and braced for impact, and did I get one, I hit the ground with a thud, no parachute roll or any grace, I was down, absolutely buzzing, the shouts of "airborne!" from the lads was great to hear, we even got to watch the boys come down after us. All the anxiety had gone, and we were left with a massive buzz which was the best feeling in the world. We almost felt superhuman. The first jump was out the way and we were elated. Beers tonight lads down the infamous Spotlight Club to celebrate.

We paraded the morning after our first jump, still buzzing, but very much still drunk from the night before.

"Fit to parachute today lads??" asked one of the PJI's, #

"yes staff!" we replied.

Were we heck! We had only finished drinking a couple of hours before! During the next couple of weeks, we had some good fortune with the weather and managed to complete a few more jumps, gradually building up our skill set. We completed jumps with equipment, which was a different challenge as before we simply wore a parachute and reserve which in real time would not make us use to anyone.

We were taught how to pack a container, which effectively is your Bergen/Backpack filled with all the equipment you need like, food, ammunition, radio equipment, med kit and dependant on your role, you may get artillery shells or mortar bombs.

Being an Airborne Soldier meant that you could be parachuting in behind enemy lines and would not be resupplied until the battle had been won. That is why we had to carry everything we would need and believe me there would be no space for lots of warm kit or sleeping bags.

Once we were shown how to build our containers, it was time to jump with it. We attached hooks and a rope to the system, with a big red (donkey's knob) handle that we would use mid-air to drop our equipment. Once again, we drilled this until we had it nailed.

Same drills, board the aircraft but this time carrying a container. Granted, this was nowhere near as heavy as it would be in the future, it was just to make sure that we could carry out the drills safely. Up we went and this time we were at 800ft so less time to fanny about. We had the usual call, "stand up fit equipment!" this time we had to fit our containers under our reserve chutes on 2 hooks. We felt like real paratroopers now, all the gear and no idea. We were to jump sim stick for this one, which meant that both sides of the aircraft would be used to dispatch us. "Port and Starboard sticks, action stations" was the cry, by this stage we had been hooked up and checked by the PJIs. Everyone knew what was coming this time, I have to say no more nerves, we knew what a buzz it is to pile out of a plane with your mates.

"Red on!", "Go", here we go again, both sides of the plane now shuffling toward those para doors, big push of the step and I'm out, this time though, there were blokes everywhere, the sky was full of Airborne Gods! Initially we seemed remarkably close to each other, but fortunately no one made contact with anyone else. We found our own little bit of clear airspace and after a check, we located our donkey nobs and gave them a big pull. Our containers left the hooks on our chest and now dangled below us on a rope that was attached to us by a karabiner. That hit the ground first and within a second, we did too.

It was an amazing feeling again and we were now so close to earning our BBCs (Blue Badge of Courage). The next jump was the one we all feared. It was to be a night decent. We did not really know what to expect, and if we were honest, we were a little bit worried about getting hurt. We prepped the same way as we did for every other jump but this time for added effect I think, we had to wear cam cream and jump with equipment to give us a real sense of things that could happen in the future.

In war time we would parachute at 250 ft with no reserve, the reason for this is to get us down quicker without the risk of us being shot to pieces on the way down. Night insertion would not be expected by the enemy either.

Here we go again, dusk when we walked out to Fat Albert and we went through the normal drills and were airborne, this time it was nice to be flying at low level over Oxfordshire and see- ing all the orange lights. We did a dummy run across the DZ and with the para doors open you could clearly see the M40 motor- way in all its glory. It gave the pilot a real good target to aim for, however get it wrong, and we would be splattered all over Mrs Miggins's windscreen.

We got the Red Light, I was very anxious now as it was once again brand-new territory, green light "go!" out we went noise of the C130 heading off into the distance and my own senses going haywire. Where is the ground? was my first question. The others around me where not a hazard and I had clear airspace so I dropped my container. You could just make out the ground at this point, but I could not really tell how high I was, so I got my feet and knees together anyway to take what was coming to me.

I now had my first experience of (Ground Rush) due to the light I must have been around 25ft from the ground, but my eyes were playing tricks and I thought I was about 50ft. As I got closer to the ground, it shot up towards me with a rapid pace and I hit the ground with a bang. I have to say it was my best jump as I was scared and tight in position ready to accept what was coming. I am now a qualified Military Parachutist or Paratrooper.

"What manner of men are these that wear the maroon beret?

They are firstly all volunteers and are toughened by physical train-ing. As a result, they have infectious optimism and that offensive eagerness which comes from well-being. They have jumped from the air and by doing so have conquered fear.

Their duty lies in the van of battle. They are proud of this honour. They have the highest standards in all things whether it be skill in battle or smartness in the execution of all peace time duties. They are in fact- men apart – every man an emperor" (Bernard Montgomery)

As above it was a huge deal to have passed not only P Company but to receive my British Parachute wings. It was a small affair for our presentation let by the OC PCAU who said lots of things which I do not really recall, but the one thing he did say which has been a massive part of my life since was,

"Welcome to the Brotherhood" this meant everything to me, I am now part of an incredibly special family (The Airborne Brotherhood) I was so proud.

CHAPTER 9

Prepare for War

I am now a trained Airborne Gunner and the next couple of months I was walking round like I owned the place, proud to be a Paratrooper and 18 years old thinking I still know it all. Life was great. I had money coming in for beer at a weekend, I played as much rugby as I wanted and still got fed if I was skint at the end of the month, life was good and after all the hard work to become a Para, being in the military was a breeze.

I remember my mum saying to me:

"Son you do realise one day you may have to go to war"?

I shrugged that off:

"No I won't don't worry about it "

Little did I realise that in a few months' time I would make their lives a living hell.

Taking it back a few notches to when I was still in training, at Strensall Ranges in Yorkshire if you remember, myself and everyone with me at the time, bared witness to an image that none of us will forget. A plane flying into the side of the World Trade Centre. This was the catalyst that would eventually send my brothers and myself to Iraq and Afghanistan.

In 2001 the US went to war in Afghanistan and some of my unit went to the capital Kabul to assist. It was the start of a long period of operations to the country, although our involvement in Afghanistan was minimal, as the good bloke that was in charge of our country at the time, Tony Blair, had other plans that were way bigger that Afghanistan at the time.

In around 2002, the UK government published a dossier on the threat posed by Iraq, stating that Sadam Hussain had Weapons of Mass Destruction (WMDS) which he could use against the West within 45 minutes of giving the order to fire. This was really frightening to hear, as we all know he had used chemical weapons on his own people, so if he had the chance, I am sure he would not hesitate to use on us! That was my thinking and how it was sold to us.

This is all we talked about with each other now for the next couple of months, do you think we will go? We were already on high readiness to deploy but we were none the wiser at this stage. The knock-on effect with all this talking was that the Regiment were upping our fitness and testing our ability to deliver under pressure. More UK exercises and there was a noticeable shake up of personnel, with movement into separate roles ensuring we had all positions covered on the Orbat, if we were to deploy on War Operations to Iraq.

My role changed now to one I was hoping to get. In my regiment we had the Gun Battery's and that was made up of Gun Crews, who deploy by parachute or helicopter and fire the guns in support of the Infantry on the ground. The other roles within the battery are a little more specialised, (gun bunnies will not like me saying this) and they are known as the Forward Observation Officer Party (FOO) or later known as the Fire Support Team (FST).

The FST main role is to direct Artillery fire and close air support (ground attack by attack aircraft) onto enemy positions whilst embedded within the infantry unit. Primarily, they are infantry soldiers, with an extended scope. The team would normally consist of a Forward Observation Officer (FOO) and a second in command (2IC) assistant known as an Ack. The other team members would include a Joint Terminal Attack Controller or (JTAC) and a Mortar Fire Controller (MFC) from the infantry unit.

As you can see, an exceedingly small specialist team that when called upon can deliver absolute devastation on the enemy with one radio call. The FST had to control all the Air Space in that area of operations and to control all the in-direct fires such as artillery and mortars. A pretty cool team to be with and would be integral on the upcoming operations.

We trained and trained over the next few months with our colleagues from the Parachute Regiment, but we were becoming very frustrated with the government as they were undecided about what role we were to take , which meant us getting fucked about. We were chomping at the bit to go to war and do what we were trained to do, and we would soon get our chance.

In February 2003 there were mass gatherings of anti- war protesters, around the world and on our doorstep in London at the prospect of a large-scale invasion of Iraq. In the background the United Nations, weapon inspectors had tried to overt this prospect and were hoping to show that Saddam did in fact have WMDs at his disposal.

The UN did not find any evidence of WMDs despite carrying out 700 plus inspections. We got the feeling that either way, we were going to end up going. The UK and US governments gave Iraq a deadline to disarm, which passed without response. With this failure, the UK and US drafted a response to the UN to which many countries apposed, such as France, Germany and Russia. No surprises there for me!

Whilst these negotiations were ongoing, we had the news that we all knew was coming. "Get the kit loaded onto the ships, make sure you have a good week on leave as from next week, we are going to Iraq!"

It really was this quick, we all knew it was coming, but still negotiations were ongoing and there may still be a resolution, we may get to Iraq and head straight home. The lads were buzzing, we are going to War! I was apprehensive as we all were deep down, but we squared everything away and went back home to have a week with our families before we were to fly out to Iraq the following week.

CHAPTER 10

The Hard Realisation

I was waiting in my mum and dad's car at Hilton Park Service Station on the M6 for my little friend Babs to pick me up. We had arranged to travel back to base together. He arrived and was full of beans and Red Bull as normal, and I gave one last hug to my Mum and shook hands with my dad. I was really upset but didn't show it as they were also being really brave and putting on a front so as not to let me see that they were suffering. They were of course. Still, none of us knew if we were going to war, or just playing along in a multinational show of force to frighten the Iraqis into submission. So, this was goodbye for now and I jumped in Babs's silver Astra. Before we left my mum said to Babs,

"Look after my boy".

That really tugged on the heartstrings and Babs, who was normally cheeky and smiling, looked them dead in the eye.

"Of course, I will, he's my brother". he answered.

He meant every word, and I for him, and him for me would do anything possible to make sure each other were OK; the trust and bond from one soldier to another, no matter what unit or background is unbreakable and one that lasts a life time. I wish this were only true later in my career. The realisation kicked in once we got back to camp. Most of the kit was now on its way to

Iraq via ship and all that we now had to do was draw our weapons, box our kit in our rooms up and get ready to roll.

The packing up of all our belongings into big MFO boxes was quite surreal. We did this in case of us being killed in action it has always been the way and the Military try to make everything as simple as possible for all eventualities. It sounds quite morbid but if I am honest, no one really cared at that point. None of us had been to war, it was all exciting to a point; we had never been shot at or ever had to shoot back. There were lots of what ifs, but at 18 we all felt invincible and as hard as a woodpecker's lips. We were not frightened and felt as if we were going on an adventure with all our mates.

RAF Brize Norton, here we come! This place held fond memories for me as it's where I qualified to parachute, but ironically it would be the place from where I would leave Blighty and potentially be the place from where I would either land back alive, or conversely, in a box. That was the reality of the situation I am afraid. Yes, you could join the military as a pilot or a chef, or even a photographer, everyone has their role and part to play, but mine along with many others was to kill any enemy that I am ordered to.

CHAPTER 11

Kuwait

We would set off from chilly England, en route to our next destination, which was Kuwait in Iraq, where we would prepare for war or get ready to come home. We gave our families a quick call and then all our mobile phones we taken off us, bagged up and we would not see them again until we flew home. Off we went, in style, on board a Royal Air Force VC10. I will be honest; it was not like flying BA or Emirates. For starters you had to fly backwards which was a little strange, and we were not presented our in-flight meal by a pretty lady with a smile. Oh no! It was chucked at us by an overweight RAF bird with a hairy top lip. What glamourous lives we led!

This aside, we all now had to mentally prepare for what was ahead. It was a confusing time, as our government still had not decided if we would go and invade Iraq or return home. It was hard to get into a killer mindset. Babs, myself, and the rest of the lads were young. I was 18 and there was a feeling of excitement more than anything else, we were going on an adventure together!

We landed in Kuwait City Airport with our body armour and helmets on. Kuwait was a friendly place, but you never know. Looking out the window, when the plane came to a stop, all we could see was sand, sand, and more sand!

We offloaded and got to a holding area where we would receive our first brief in country however, it was too fucking hot to listen! I had never experienced anything like the heat there, it must have been around 30 degrees, which may not sound a lot, but it was a definite shock to the system. It was extremely dry, and we could not get enough water into our systems.

It was now the 5th March 2003 and we were staying in top notch tented accommodation which was great. We had fresh food, cot beds and protection from the elements which was all we needed. We could sense that everything was still building up for us to cross the border into Iraq, but no definitive order was forthcoming. During the next few weeks, we had to get our training up to speed. That would include zeroing our SA80 Rifles on a range to ensure that our groupings were correct enough to hit the enemy, we also had to prepare to be attacked with biological and chemical weapons by the Iraqi Army.

This for me was the scariest bit. Going back to AFC Harrogate we had our first taste of chemical warfare in the CS test chamber, or as we all called it, THE GAS CHAMBER! If you have ever served in the military or are thinking about joining, the gas chamber is a moment in your life you will never forget.

Our Nuclear, Biological, Chemical (NBC) equipment was horrendous to wear. It consisted of an S10 Respirator with interchangeable filters, charcoal lined smock and trousers, boots, and gloves. Along with this we had to carry out different drill's dependant on the situation and we would get hammered with these drills in training with the call, GAS! GAS! GAS! We would then have literally seconds to fit our respirators to our faces and blow out, ourselves shouting Gas! Gas! Gas! It was imperative that we were skilled in this in real life if we could mask up in 5 seconds, that was enough time for the chemical, biological, or nuclear agent to penetrate our respiratory system and kill us instantly. On top of wearing this kit that would fatigue us, we could have to potentially fight for hours in it too, for Paratroopers nothing is impossible.

So as young recruits we lined up outside the CS gas chamber ready to be tested on our drills. The chamber was filled with CS gas. This chemical, although not deadly, causes stress on the body and acts as an incapacitant. We were all fully kitted up outside the chamber and were called into the smoke-filled chamber, although we had respirators on, we could smell the CS which was not a great sign, but it had no effect on us. One by one, we were told that we had to remove our respirators and then say our name, rank, and number, then we could leave. Simple I thought, I will be out of here in no time. I was first, I was anxious:

"Bentley take your respirator off and give me the information required to leave the chamber".

This would be a piece of cake I thought. I grabbed the bottom of my respirator, took a big deep breath, closed my eyes and lifted off my respirator and stated –

"Corporal I am 25123908, Private Bentley Corporal!"

In my mind I had passed the test, or so I thought, until the corporal asked me "What's your mum's name "?

I was not expecting this, and I took a breath in and it was game over, my throat was burning, my eyes pouring, and I felt like I could not breath. I was gone, and I could not function. I was wrenching and I then started to panic. In the panic I instinctively started to flail out and get a little punchy before I got a slap off the Corporal the door opened, and I was out in the fresh air. If you have seen the movie Platoon where Willem Dafoe comes out the jungle having been shot several times, falls to his knees with his arms in the air. This was me, gasping for breath, with snot and tears pouring down my face, I didn't want to go through that ever again.

During our brief stay in Kuwait we experienced one of the worst sandstorms in the country's history, it was like a warning of what was to come.

CHAPTER 12

Going to War

We got the nod, it was on! On the 18th March 2003, in the House of Commons it was voted that military action was needed in order to rid the Saddam regime of its power to use WMDs against the rest of the world. We were called together and told the news that we would hope would come.

We were all paraded on some thick wooden decking, inside a red-hot crowded tent along with all the rest of the Battery, wondering what was in store for us. Wiggling our toes in our crappy issued desert boots, trying to stop our feet from going numb, we stood and listened to our Battery Commander (BC) and other senior ranks give us their best pep talk. We were right next to the scoff house and could smell chips cooking, which reminded me of home, but then, the occasional blast of the portaloos as people were going backwards and forwards for a dump.

"We are going to War men!" words that I thought I would not here all that time ago at the Army Careers Office. We had our orders and was told to get all our weapons re-zeroed, the necessary vehicles ready and to get our personal affairs in order. Get our affairs in order? Sounds a little morbid that, I am not going to die! I am sure we all had that outlook and there was few in the regiment that had seen combat before, so it was new to us all.

The one thing we did have to do, which not many 18-year-old lads do in normal times, was write our wills.

I was thinking to myself, what if I was killed? What I have I got that my parents would get if I were killed? I had nothing to show for my 3 years of service so far. Every penny I had went on beer and we used to get pissed up every night of the week. We would wake up pissed, do PT pissed and then the only time we were sober was lunch time. I did not have a penny to my name at the end of the month, but we always knew that we would have food and accommodation free of charge.

Battle prep was now in full flow, weapon systems zeroed, we were issued our equipment, radios, ammunition, and rations for the first few days of the war. Some of the equipment we were issued with we were not used to having back in the UK.

I was a little uneasy when I was issued 3 Combo pens. These were for us to use on ourselves if we came under attack from Nuclear, Biological or Chemical weapons, after all that's the reason we were going to war; to stop Saddam attacking people with these types of weapons. We were to push these Combo pens onto our thighs and press the top, which would then shoot a 5cm needle into our legs, delivering Atropine and Pralidoxime into our systems to counteract the effects of these weapons. I did not want to be doing this to myself. We were also issued Nerve Agent Pre-Treatment Set (NAPS) tablets that we would soon be ordered to take.

So let's talk NAPS. I wish I could say that it stood for taking a little break in the day to shut your eyes and relax, no, these tablets we were ordered to take in case of a chemical attack. I say ordered, and that meant standing on parade, physically taking a tablet, putting it in our mouths, swallowing it and then letting a senior ranking officer check inside our mouth to make sure we took it! We had no say in this, it was a direct order and we had no clue what if any side effects would be. The tablets held Pyridostigmine Bromide which for your information is a cholinesterase inhibitor. The tablets were supposed to counteract the effects of some nerve agent and we were ordered to take them as there was a considerable risk of us coming under attack as we entered Iraq. This was scary; getting shot at I thought I could handle, but getting gassed?

Two morphine auto injectors were issued to all of us and that was the end of the scary kit, now for the good stuff. Normally back home on the range we would be issued with about 60 rounds or bullets as you may call them. It was hugely different now; we were prepping to engage an enemy so all a sudden we had kit flying at us from every direction.

I was issued around 200 rounds of 5.56 NATO ammunition for my personal weapon, SA80 rifle, 2 HE L109A1 grenades, smoke grenades and a Schmooley (illumination rocket). A kid in a sweet shop comes to mind, I felt like John J Rambo.

CHAPTER 13

The Invasion

We were ready to rock and got into our teams as part of the 3 Para Battlegroup. We loaded our non-armoured, soft skin land rover and trailer in preparation to cross the border from Kuwait into Iraq.

We had some cracking blokes in our FST, Captain Jarmon, Rob, Pritch and Ringo. As I was still way down the pecking order along with Ringo, we had to cram ourselves into the rear of the Landover for the foreseeable, which was not comfortable at all, every bump in the desert you would land on a piece of comms equipment, bang your head on the roof or get something sharp digging into your arse cheek. We were going to war, so this was the least of our worries.

Now for a bit of history. On 19th March 2003, the Gun Batterys of my Regiment, 7th Parachute Regiment, RHA fired the first shots of the war by any coalition ground troops as they moved forward with the U.S. Marine Corps, this is always a sore subject between us members of a FST and the Gun crews as we were meant to be the forward observers and the Guns remaining behind. This time roles were reversed but I am glad they got to engage the enemy first and clear the way for the infantry and Tanks later.

On the 20th March 2003, the invasion began. It started with an aerial bombardment of suspected buildings in the capital Bagh-dad where it was thought Saddam Hussain was meant to be liv-ing. Later it turned out that he had not visited the site since 1995, good intelligence hey?

We slowly made our way from our base in Kuwait up to the border of Iraq, I remember feeling excited, not scared, and ready to pull the trigger if needed. It was dusty and noisy up towards the border and all we could smell was toxic fumes of oil being burnt.

We approached the crossing into Iraq, nothing glamorous, just an engineer bridge and a pissed off looking Military Policeman stood marshalling across. I hated the Military Police and could never understand why you would join the Army to be a knob and arrest your own. However later the Royal Military Police would face one of the largest losses of life of the war.

We got the order to make ready, which meant that we had to ensure all our personnel weapon systems were good to go in case of enemy action. We already had a magazine of 30 rounds or bullets loaded on to our weapon systems, the make ready meant that we checked our safety catch, change lever was in semi-automatic function, sights test and then with our left hand, over our right we grabbed the cocking handle, worked the parts back to front and gave a forward assist to ensure that there was now a round in the chamber and ready for use.

For all you weapon buffs our standard issue personal weapon system at the time was a The SA80A1 assault rifle (L85A1) which entered service in 1985, replacing the venerable L1A1 SLR (7.62x51mm NATO) as the British military's standard as-sault rifle. Chambered in 5.56x45mm NATO, with a magazine capacity of 30 rounds, the SA80A1's ammunition was less powerful but lighter and easier to carry in high quantities than its predecessor. Most front-line SA80A1s were fitted with SUSAT (Sight Unit Small Arms Trilux) scopes, with 4x magnifi-cation, making for an accurate, albeit heavy weapon.

I was not a bad shot at all, and the effective accurate range of this weapon system was 300-400 metres. It may not sound a long distance but accurate enough to hit an enemy soldier from distance or to keep their heads down long enough for us to get up close and make it a little more personal.

Crossing the border was awfully slow going and it was our task as 16 Air Assault Brigade to secure all the oil refineries around Rumailia. These refineries were of strategic importance and we had to secure them before they were destroyed by Saddam's forces. If you remember any footage of the Iraq War these refineries were always on the news as the majority were set on fire by the Iraq Forces before we could get to them.

As I said earlier, it was terribly slow going for us in the vehicles and every time we stopped, we had to jump out and start digging shell scrapes in case of bombardment by the enemy. This although was really hard work paid off later. We had our shovels and started to dig trenches in the rock-hard ground and baking heat, losing fluid as quickly as we could drink it. We all knew the scale of the threat and were always prepared for the Iraqis to use biological or chemical agents on us. I remember thinking that if there was a right time to get us with it, now's the time, as we had just invaded.

CHAPTER 14

<u>Incoming!!!!</u>

O ur first day entering Iraq and the shells began to fall, we had the cry "GAS GAS GAS" which to this day sends a shiver down my spine. We had incoming enemy shells landing within 100 meters of our vehicles and all we could do was take cover. We could not see who was attacking us but all we knew was that it might be gas. I think whoever gave the order for us all to wear full Romeo dress state was nuts and just flapping but sweating with our S10 respirators on just added to all the confusion of the situation.

The bombardment stopped and to be honest none of us were killed or injured but it was the first real taste of what was to come. Digging holes and sweating our bollocks off wearing full NBC gear was the name of the game, no fighting the enemy, heat and exhaustion was the biggest killer at the time.

We found out later that day that it was a mixture of artillery, mortars and tank rounds being aimed in our direction, the worst of the fire coming at us from D30s which was a 122mm Howitzer. The incoming soon stopped as our guns fired back with an 18 Gun Fire Mission and absolutely malleted the lot with precision, neutralising the enemy, disabling their equipment, and breaking morale. They said in WW2 that even if the shells did not land in the trenches to kill the enemy, the constant noise and the confusion of the bombardment were enough to break their will. I can recognise this and although we faced nothing like the soldiers of WW2, we were the ones dishing it out to the Iraqis and we would soon see that it did the job.

So far we had a little bit of resistance, nothing major and a few of the guys had contact with the enemy, 2 days in and I had not even seen the so called enemy, nothing but sand and the end of my shovel whilst digging holes. It was not like the films and I look back now and think that it was not too bad at all, however that being said Afghanistan later in the story was a little different.

We were now about 20 km into Iraq from the Kuwait border, and we got to Rumalia bridge which crossed the river Euphrates, a very historical and religious part of the world and was an area within the biblical Garden of Eden.

We will touch on my faith a little later, but as we were about to roll out over the bridge, the heavens opened, and we had the worst rainstorm in Iraq for the last 20 years. We were not prepared for it we had vehicles getting bogged in, water leaking all over our comms equipment. It was insane, it felt like the Gods were halting our advance in the Iraqis favour.

Some hours later we had dried out a little and we advanced over the bridge. There was quite a delay due to the number of traps set for us by the enemy forces that had to be dealt with. They had set IEDs up, trip wires and set charges on all the doors on top of the bridge buildings.

In my 18 years so far, I had not lost any family members, been in any nasty accidents, seen anyone who had been killed and the day had come. We crossed the bridge and I counted 4 dead Iraqis, they were scattered across the bridge and looked as if they had been in defensive positions awaiting our arrival. It was hard to tell how they had been killed. One I recall being face down by the side of a wall, wearing blue overalls, could not see his face, another was sat up against the wall, eyes open, ashen in colour and in an unnatural position. I will never forget his face. It was a shock to the system for me to process however I was surprised at the lack of blood and guts, there was no smell, no weapons and just empty shells of people who were alive and now are not.

Thoughts entered my head that someone had killed these people, could I do that? We would have to see. It did not upset me but as the others laughed and joked "ha-ha get that you Iraq bastard" I could not help thinking that it was not right and proper to mock them. Yes, they are an enemy and what had to be done however they were dead and that now it, move on.

As some people say, the dead soldiers could have been fathers, husbands, brothers etc, none of that bothered me one bit, if they were in the way and wanted to fight. It was either them or us.

Following the crossing we took some more incoming shelling, this time a little closer and a bit more frightening. It was artillery from an Iraq battery, and they had obviously set the shells to airburst over the top of us. We had to dive under the vehicles as that was the only protection available to us at the time. Once again, we could not see the firing point or have any clue where we were getting attached from, this was so frustrating for us.

A few days rolled on, with some patrolling on the ground around local villages until we came across hundreds of people waving a white flag.

They were Iraq soldiers and before we had the chance to take them on, it appeared that they all had surrendered to us. They looked dishevelled and not interested in fighting us in the slightest. They did not appear to be professionals and it soon became clear that they were very scared.

My team was tasked to take a group of Iraq soldiers to disarm and search for them for intelligence. This was a nervous time for me as it was the first time, I had had to deal with anything like this and how I would act would be the key. As paratroopers it could be said that we were naturally aggressive but on the other side of that, highly professional. We were their captors and although they clearly had given up, I did not want to come across placid and start giving them hugs. One at a time we took their weapons off them and piled them up. I recall having my weapon pointed at them all the time, not in an aggressive posture however in such a position that I could let a few rounds off directly at them if needed.

I have to say it felt good, and I felt in control. The majority of the Prisoners Of War (POW) were very compliant but there were a couple who were clearly officers who felt they ought to be treated a little differently. Not happening - they all got treated the same. An officer came through and it was his turn to be searched. He had cleaner uniform than the rest, clearly ate more than the rest and had a pretty well-groomed tash. He took exception to me pointing my weapon at him and with his right hand, grabbed the end of my barrel and in an aggressive manner pushed it away whilst at the same time, gobbing off at me in his local dialect.

My officer and my team looked at me to say, what you going to do Benny? I did what I thought right at the time and cracked him right in the jaw with the butt of my rifle. He went down like a toilet seat, blood pouring from his mouth. I have to say if I was him I would of probably done the same, he was showing defiance in front of his men, however following my actions I held out my arm and helped him back up, he straightened himself out gave me a nod and followed the others.

Was what I did necessary? I still believe so, and it had the desired effect. I feel it could have escalated had I gone with a softer approach, we live and learn. This was my first contact with the enemy, and it had not gone as I thought it would when I was on P COY training to be this controlled killer. We were professional and treated the prisoners with respect and dignity just as long as they behaved.

The war rolled on from the 20th March to the 1st May and in that time, there were casualties and fatalities on our side, but thankfully none from our units. If you remember back earlier in the story, I spoke about SGT TC one of my rugby coaches whilst at Harrogate. Sadly, he was the first British Soldier to die in the 2003 Iraq War. What made it worse was that he was slotted by one of his own men. He was struggling with a protester and was fatally shot; this really was sad news for me especially the way it was done.

The other major blow was the loss of life suffered by the Royal Military Police who were killed by a mob in Majar al-Kabir, southern Iraq, on 24 June 2003 following the war.

The only 2 other major actions we had during the War phase was to secure the Gas Oil Separation Plants (GOSPS) which were of strategic importance (probably for the oil) in my opinion going forward, we met zero resistance to our occupation of these facilities and the biggest threat would come from the fumes and the structure of the buildings themselves.

The only time I got to do what I was trained to do came when our team was tasked to break away from 3 Para to support the Pathfinders Platoon. This was exciting for me and I was chuffed to be involved. We would be going out on a mobile patrol to get engaged by the enemy so that we could strike back and clear the area of the remain enemy elements. The Pathfinder Platoon acts as the brigade's advance force and reconnaissance force. Its role includes finding and marking drop zones and helicopter landing zones for air landing operations. Once the main force has landed, the platoon supplies tactical intelligence and offensive action roles for the brigade. They were in my mind the best of the Paras and it was great to get out on the ground with them.

We headed out patrolling from our GOSP in Rumalia and it did not take long for us to run into trouble. We came under contact from a Light Anti-Tank Weapon which just missed the Pathfinders vehicle in front of us. This time we could see the bastards who were shooting at us and the Pathfinders started putting some 50-calibre machine gun down onto the enemy positions. There was sporadic small arms fire, possible AK47 7.62 rounds snapping over our heads. It was crazy and really got the heart pumping, after all this time it felt like we were at war, not with the heat, or equipment, but with the enemy.

It was our team's turn to step up and get to work. We stood on the tailgate of our vehicle and Pritch spotted a threat through his binoculars. About 800 meters away there was an Iraq ZSU 24 Air Defence Battery. They are self-propelled armoured vehicles with obvious 4 23 mm cannons mounted on the front with a satellite dish on the rear. Pritch was a guru at vehicle recognition, and I had to agree. We could see through the binoculars that there were 4 vehicles manoeuvring into position to engage us. Through the blurry heated desert, we could see the diesel smoke coming from their engines, so we had to act quickly.

The boss gave the command and we sent our first Fire Mission of the war to our Gun line. "Fire Mission Battery" grid, altitude and direction were given with the description of the target. Armoured ZSU battery in the open PD 5 rounds fire for effect! This was awesome; we had just called for 20 rounds of high explosive 105 mm artillery shells to strike the enemy. We had the gun line call ready on the target. I was given the command of FIRE! From my officer. "Fire Over" we sent, and we again waited for the gun's reply. "shot over" we heard in the distance the rumbling of 4 light guns unleashing hell, like thunder and then the sound of a whhhhooooosh over the top of us. "Rounds complete over" I replied.
"Rounds complete out!
We looked into the target area and waited for the artillery to land.

It was spot on pretty much and we could see smoke and fire coming from the vehicles, we also saw 2 people running away. After a few minutes, the dust settled, and the fires raged. There was no more vehicular movement, but there was without doubt enemy soldiers in the area that were trying to help their comrades.

We did our Battle Damage Assessment and we felt that we had not done enough to successfully disable their capabilities so we gave another order to our guns, this time changing the method to air burst in order to hit the troops in the open. This would give them a taste of how we felt when they did it to us however, they put 3 or 4 over our heads and we were about to give them 20 of Her Majesty's finest. We pushed the rounds 100m further back this time and we could here again the rounds overhead and watched again for the rounds to land. As expected, there was shells air bursting 18 meters above the ground. As the dust settled, we looked again and there was no more movement and we were satisfied that we had neutralised the threat.

We had just neutralised the enemy and disabled their equipment. People always ask soldiers, "have you ever killed anyone?" it is the worst thing that you could ask. It is not sexy like the films at times, I was not running towards the enemy with a bayonet fitted ready to thrust it into another man's chest. There were no feelings of regret for me, but there would have been if we had not of done what we had done, they could have potentially taken our one of our aircraft or ground assets. It was not personal it was a job and one done well with precision accuracy.

Later, we were told that there were up to 10 plus dead enemy soldiers on that position. They had the chance to leave or surrender but they stood fast and held their ground and credit to them for this. although it was a strange, surreal feeling I had inside the pit of my stomach, I knew that I had done what I had meant to do, none of my friends were injured and we had potentially saved others with our actions.

This was my first and only involvement with the enemy the entire time of the Iraq war. Later, in Afghanistan it would not be my last encounter with an enemy force.

The Iraq war was uneventful from then on, we soon changed from a war fighting role to a peace support mission. As a battlegroup we were not severely affected by the war other than taking a load of drugs to protect us from chemical and biological attack, which did not happen. We had minimal contact with the enemy and an incredibly low casualty rate in the grand scheme of things. We slowly got the local Iraq population to come out of hiding and resume a normal pattern of life.

In a nutshell there were lots of firsts for me out in Iraq, first exposure to the desert, first glimpse of death, first encounter with an enemy, all be that on their surrender and our fire mission on the ZSU battery that took the lives of up to 20 people. The threat was out there, and I believe there was an element of luck in it all. I was not afraid as a young 18-year-old Paratrooper and it was exciting, but it could have been hugely different.

We returned home as heroes following a 6-month operational tour of duty. Did I feel like a hero? Not at all! Do I feel that we made a difference in the world? not really! and would I go again? Of course, and that is for one reason alone, my mates!

Just to put other people's perspectives into this story, I mentioned that I put my mum and dad through Hell when I was away on operations in Iraq and Afghanistan. At the time I could manage due to being there in the present and knowing what was going on, but people back home must have been worried sick.

My mum and dad never spoke of how they felt until recently when I asked them to write down their thoughts. My dad could not but my mum did, and I felt horrendous after reading it.

"I hate bonfire night, I was stood outside with Dave hearing the boom, boom of the fireworks", "it sounded a bit like this mum" Dave said. "I have never been to a firework display since. I have never felt pain like it when Dave went to war, Iraq first, then Afghanistan, it tore me apart. I find it so hard to talk about that time in my life, I cried constantly, I watched and recorded every hour of sky news, I had hundreds of hours of tapes that I watched over and over, just trying to get a glimpse of my son.

My mental health suffered, I had severe anxiety episodes, I was sleep walking, pulling drawers and wardrobes apart throwing everything everywhere, not knowing anything until I walked into his room the next day. I had to seek help from my GP, he thought the searching through the drawers etc was my subconscious looking for my boy, I would wake up sweating, scared having nightmares and palpitations and very occasionally I still do.

I thought I was going mad. My GP believed I was suffering with PTSD, I could not be, I had never heard of it.

I worked at the time as an Emergency Controller for West Midlands Ambulance Service and during the conflicts I oversaw the repatriation of servicemen and women who arrived back in the

UK. They flew into Birmingham airport then were transferred to Selly Oak Hospital for further treatment. I remember Dave's friend Ben Parkinson's name pop up on the screen and I fell to pieces, I knew him! Dave's mate from the regiment. I could no longer do this role. At the time Ben Parkinson was the most severely injured surviving soldier since WW2. I cried for him and his family and just wanted Dave home".

I still cry and am doing so now writing this, I hate thinking of those days, I hate the pictures, the music that reminds me of that time, I cannot watch anything that reminds me of that time. Nothing with soldiers, war, or anything to do with Iraq and Afghanistan.

So many of Dave's friends were killed or severely, injured, there was and still is so much pain, how can I describe that time? I cannot.

Suffering with (Mums guilt) how can I? my boy came home, thank God, a lot did not, and I still feel their pain. I have kept all my guilt, thoughts and wishes all wrapped up in a box, hidden right at the back of my mind. I must put them all back in the box again now.

I love you Dave and I am so proud of you in everything you have achieved. (Glennis Bentley)

CHAPTER 15

Back Home

O nce we got home it was very strange, apart from worrying my parents to death I was happy, or so I thought. We had money saved up from the tour, the kudos of returning from Iraq as heroes, we had it all, however something was missing.

When we got back to the UK, we cleaned our kit and went on leave. There was no decompression package. What I mean by that, there was no time for us to reflect on what we had been through as a group the previous 6 months. The reality was that we were lucky, and we got away with things, but I have no doubt that I and others were secretly suffering inside.

Looking back at myself and my actions and talking to my parents, my behaviour had completely changed from previously deploying to Iraq. Looking back now I know I was incredibly angry, short tempered and had a chip on my shoulder. I would drink as much alcohol as I could until I vomited or passed out. This was not a normal behaviour of a normal lad my age from where I was brought up. At the time I could see no problem, but I was constantly in trouble and always fighting.

Following our leave, we all returned to our unit and it was clear to see that I was not alone in this pattern of behaviour. We stood on parade and no word of a lie there were about 70 percent of the lads that either had black eyes or split lips, this clearly should have been a sign to the seniors that we were all having issues.

The Battery Sergeant Major (BSM) – Scary man stood Infront of us and asked us a series of questions. "Who is skint, put your hands up!", 90 percent of us put our hands up, we must have saved around 6 grand on tour and what did I have to show for it? You guessed it, nothing! "who has been in trouble with the police? Put your hands up" the odds were slightly better, roughly 50 percent. All for fighting and looking back now I know why.

Most of us had not been on an operational tour before, we were young and hungry to see action. We were all paratroopers and we were all trained to kill the enemy, no dressing it up, that is fact! We were not vets or doctors or pilots in the Royal Air Force, we were soldiers in the fighting Army. Now this said I do not condone violence and random violent acts on anyone, however in my opinion now looking back, we all had factual issues that were not addressed as we returned from a war fighting mission.

We were fully prepared to go to War take life or pay the ultimate sacrifice for the queen but more importantly than that for our mates. Some months later I fell on the wrong side of the law and although I am not making excuses for the following actions, I really truly believe that it was due in part to the effects and experiences I went through on tour in Iraq.

We plodded along in the regiment for the next few months, conducting training exercises and other bits and bobs but 2004/2005 really was not my year. During these 2 years I was charged and convicted in 2 separate criminal acts that would disgrace and embarrass me for years to come. As I said earlier without making excuses what I did looking back was very wrong and I will regret to my dying day however I do feel that there was certainly an element of trauma I along with others were still dealing with.

Right at the start of the story I told you I loved a fight and was a bit of a rogue, this was all well and good but I didn't really leave anyone with any permanent damage or life time trauma, it was school boy stuff. Alcohol as we know does not help matters if you have a short fuse and the dreaded wife beater (Stella) was not the best choice to drink regularly.

The start of my criminality was in a safe space at my local rugby club. We played a game and as normal we would drink our body weight in beer, sing songs and wake up in the morning with a bad head. This time it was not to be. As sometimes that happens when a group of lads get drunk it gets quite eventful, however a scuffle broke out near the entrance to the club and there was a fair few lads piling in to each other, looking back now I should of walked away and had nothing to do with it, however as I said I was having really issues going on that I was not really aware of.

I waded in punched one lad, then another, got punched a few times myself and knocked to the floor, kicked, and punched on the ground until I managed to get myself up. Feeling a little groggy as I recall I was then approached by a big lad who was obviously going to cause me some damage, by this time the scuffle was a full on riot and people where punching and kicking people all over the shop. The big fella who came at me chased me around the other side of the bar. Without a backward step I punched him on the jaw, and he went down with a thud, right into a set of spirit optics, which regretfully now cut him quite badly. This was not the end of the story. I went back to my parents' house to sleep it all off but the following morning there was a knock on the door.

David Bentley one of the police officers asked, that is me I replied. I knew what was coming, David you are under arrest on suspicion of Actual Bodily Harm, you do not have to say anything..........

Oh, dear the bloke that I had punched in the bar brawl at my local Rugby club, turned out to be an off-duty Policeman. Great I had now been arrested and charged with ABH. War hero to zero in a throw of a fist. I was taken to the local police station in Cannock and was processed as they say. I had an interview with a couple of officers, and I made their work easy, I did not try to pass the blame, make excuses I just told it as it was. I knew I had fucked up but if anything has served me well throughout my time, it is telling the truth. An age-old tradition that your mum and dad would have instilled in you. It was not great for me at the time and I deserved everything I got however a bit of advice for you in any situation or role you find yourselves in later in life, just tell the truth, it is far more beneficial than going in circles, you will also get more respect, that is fact.

I had photos taken of my fists which were marked up, I had a photo taken and fingerprints. I had mouth swabs done, all of which meant I was on the criminal database even before I went to court.

I was bailed and waited for a court appearance which would take place at Staffordshire Magistrates Court. I dressed smartly, had a shave, and turned up to court nice and early. I was met by the duty solicitor who would try and defend me, there was no point as I would own up to my actions anyway. I felt nervous to see what would happen to me but worse than that I felt embarrassed that I had let myself and my family down. I did not feel bad for the bloke I punched and to this day still do not, he was a police officer and that was his get out of jail card, I got stitched up. That aside I stood in the dock and pleaded guilty as charged, I would now await my punishment.

As this was my first offence I was given 150 hours of community service and a £500 fine, what a bastard!!!!, from now on every Sunday I would have to pay back in the community with a load of other scrotal bags just like me.

Every Sunday I had to turn up at my local community centre and paint bird boxes, humiliating, I didn't mind the painting if I am honest but what I minded was I had to complete my hours in the company of some right dossers who clearly are regulars on the community service circuit. In my thinking, yes I had done wrong, but had no support whatsoever returning from War in Iraq, I was a veteran and faced things many hadn't in everyday life, I felt worthless and exactly the same as the dossers I was working alongside.

I remember one of them asked me a question, just like the films, "what you in for" my reply "fuck off else I will throat chop you" as you can see the punishment was not helping me learn to control my temper or put to bed the demons starting to build up in my head.

CHAPTER 16

Welcome to the Jungle

We shot off to Kenya now for a few months which was a welcome change on exercise, beautiful country with great training opportunities and the chance to unwind on r and r. we stayed in Nanuki which in military circles is very popular for cheap Tusker beer and other entertainment that is for another story. We had a wonderful time over there, and we worked hard in training and had opportunities to relax and unwind from it all. We went on safari and climbed Mount Kenya, which was utterly amazing, we got to chillout in a few lodges and just generally enjoy our time. I do believe that it was needed to get our heads back in the game and recharge our batteries from such a strange 6 months out in Iraq.

It wasn't all fun and games out in Kenya, the heat and terrain in a place called Archers Post or as we called it Archers Roast was hard going, it is located near the Equator and when fighting through the trees and soldiering you really needed to be on top of your personal admin to stay fit.

On my Team out there was Captain Pete Beaumont from Stoke, Taff Seaward from port Talbot and you guessed it, Babs. Great bunch of blokes and we had lots of fun and lots of heart to hearts. I mentioned earlier we trained in a place called Archers Post, it was the hottest place on earth, poor Babs had some ginger in him and had to constantly smother the sunscreen on himself to prevent him cooking. I remember the one day we were doing some, close quarter battle (CQB) drills through some jungle terrain. It was mine and Babs turn to go through, we both had separate lanes for safety with people behind us to ensure that there were no accidents.

I spotted my first target and engaged it, "contact front" I screamed. I squeezed off a couple of rounds in the general direction, found some appropriate cover, into a bastard bush as we called them, squeezed off another 5 or 6 rounds, checked my ammunition pouches and got ready to charge at the target switching to automatic fire as I did.

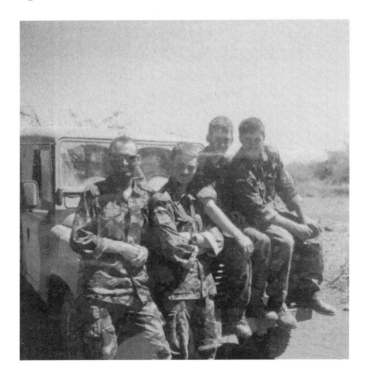

(left to right, Pete, Taff, Babs and me in Archers Post Kenya)

I had just switched to automatic ready to start brassing up the target and then from nowhere appeared Babs like a man possessed, screaming and running out the trees shooting my target like Rambo, he nearly fuckin killed me. To this day he said he saw where I was, but those bullets were zipping passed my head with pace and a couple even dropped Infront of my feet so I am not sure, we did have an argument a few nights before, so I guess we will never know. "Watch where you are firing you fucking idiot" I shouted, "that was too close!", "miles away from you" he chuckled in his manc accent.

I referred to bastard bushes earlier and a funny story about them. me, Pete Taff and Babs were patrolling through the bush, which was really hard going in the baking sun, sweating, thirsty, irritable we all cracked on. Pete used to say that I was like an elephant plodding through the trees, not very tactical. We ended up getting caught in a bastard bush ambush, I would have rather been in a minefield at the time, they were bloody everywhere. These bushes had thorns on them the size of shark's teeth, they were horrible. I remember I fell forward into one and one pierced my skin in between my second and third knuckle and hit the bone in my hand. The pain was excruciating, and it was pouring with blood. I cleaned it out best as I could with water and iodine, but it was not good enough. A day later my hand was like an elephant's foot. We were operating by a hill called Kamanga. The lads having no sympathy called me Kamanga Hand for the rest of the tour. Being an airborne soldier meant that I could not just walk to the med centre and get it seen, I had to wait a further 2 days before I could get it sorted. I had a temperature; my hand was infected and red, I was hallucinating, and I struggled to fire my weapon, but the key thing was that I could still soldier on, and although uncomfortable it was bearable. Gritted my teeth and got the job done and was not a burden on the lads.

Back to camp, IV antibiotics and it was sorted. A really tough environment to operate in and similar to Brunei where I take you next briefly to discuss an issue we had within our team with a bad egg of an officer.

Another Jungle but a prevalent story from my time in Brunei, which I wanted to mention from a team perspective. I was now second in command of an FST and we had a new officer joining the team who was young, keen and tried ridiculously hard to get on. He was what we called in the trade, A Massive Bell End. He was not a leader or in fact a team player and I clashed with him constantly. He was not speaking to us or involving us in any of the planning, which is key in such a tight nit Team, he would wander around looking like a bag of shit and get the younger lads to fill up his water bottles and do his errands, a real tosser. One day he threw his water bottles to me whilst he was lay chilling on his bed. "Bentley go and fill these up for me, there's a good chap", I was fuming and taught him a lesson that day. I took them back to my block and filled them both up with piss, I filled one up myself but didn't have enough in the tank to fill the other so I got one of the lads to do it for me. "you have pissed in these" I am going to speak with the BSM" he did too the snitch and although I got a bollocking he didn't get me to fill them again. Moving on we had lots of issues but we headed into our final attack exercise and I had tried to put him under my wing, although he was an officer I wanted to look after him and impart some knowledge and experience on to him. He had none of it and clearly thought I was talking bollox.

It was hot, humid sticky and hard going in the final attack. As mentioned, before it was our job as an FST to stay up with the lead infantry sections so that we could provide them in-direct artillery fire. I could see captain nob head start to struggle physically and advised him to sit his arse down before he falls down, well similar words to that affect, he wouldn't have it and tried to be a hero and crack on. Minutes later, man down, man down, that was it, he hit the deck like a toilet seat and was incapable of doing anything. He was salivating at the mouth, making incomprehensible noises and it was down to us the junior members of the Team to sort him out.

We lay him down and took all his equipment off and soaked him with water, we put up a basher to keep him out the sun and called a company medic over. He was obviously acutely dehydrated and suffering heat illness. I had to take command of the

Team and whilst doing my job for the infantry lads, suppression the enemy with artillery I had to also get a casevac organised to get this doughnut out of the jungle.

Although it was a training environment in Brunei, similar to Kenya, it was very real in the way we trained as the old saying goes, train hard fight easy, is the way we did things.

The company medic sorted him out and we managed to get a helicopter in for him and he was later flown back to the med centre.

We finished our exercise and we got good kudos from the battery commander for our actions, but I was not happy I had a bone to pick with our officer.

I went to see him once back at the barracks and he was up and about which was good to see, however I was going to rip him a new arsehole for the way he had conducted himself throughout the tour he stopped me speaking and said, "I apologise for how I have been, I was too keen to succeed and in doing so I put our team at risk and our mission at risk "words to that affect, he acknowledged that he had messed up, he apologised to the rest of the team and from this we were able to move forward with a bit more trust.

We looked after him like a brother in the heat of battle and to this day he will never forget this. what I have learnt in all my years of being in Teams is to listen to all, get everyone's views and opinions and you will have better outcomes. It does not matter if you are a CEO of a multimillion-pound company or a bin man, you need to involve others and without the Team we are nothing. I have had some fantastic officers in my time but this one was awful, and had it been at War he would have compromised us all.

CHAPTER 17

Round 2, seconds out

We got back to the UK again and the same as before had some money in our pockets and chips on our shoulders again. Me and a few lads headed out into Reading for a night out, jeans on, desert boots and puffer jackets at the ready. Already full to the brim of Stella we headed into town and tried a few bars and drank a few more and then a few more, looking back it was ridiculous and I do not know how we were able to stand but this is when our training became very dangerous.

We were in a night club now probably early morning after drinking heavily for several hours, we had money to splash out and there were about 5 of us left. We were getting some attention from the local ladies which did not seem to be going down with the local males, they were clearly out for trouble and were intimidated by us, although we were not interested in them at all.

It began as always with a War of words and some pushing and shoving inside the night club. Tensions rising the door staff soon had a job on their hands to get us all out the club, they tried to be a little rough with us as they clearly knew we were soldiers, dressed up in stone wash jeans and desert boots. We got outside and the fresh air hit us all, which made things a little clearer.

The bunch of lads who were getting at us in the nightclub returned with a few more members to take us on. Once again in hindsight we should have acknowledged there was going to be trouble and left the area. We did not leave the area and a mass brawl ensued. The lads and I were getting attacked from all angles by 10-12 lads. Punches and bottles flying in as we looked to defend ourselves. We did just that, we stayed together and got out of trouble with pretty minor injuries.

The scary bit was to come, both scared for our lives but more so scared what we could do to other people. Drink fuelled and frustration from our tour in Iraq, we were fired up and were dangerous weapons. The fighting stopped and we headed off to return to our barracks, however not knowing the local area so well we were cut off once again by these local lads. This time they did not just have fists and bottles, they had knives and metal poles.

They came at us in one last ditch attempt to inflict some damage to us, but what they did not expect is for us all to face the danger and attack back head on. This may read like I am trying to sex up a situation, it's not for effect I am just trying to highlight the situation at the time and what we did to get out of it, later on you will see what detrimental effects these incidents had on my career.

With knives drawn and metal bars swinging, I remember getting hit on top of my head and feeling like someone was pouring hot water on my head. This is fact was blood and my head were bleeding profusely. There was lots of lashing around as they tried to stab us with the small blades they had in their possession. We disarmed them, overpowered them and they fled away up the road. We were lucky, but I was surprised that all this had gone on and there was not a sign of the police. Had they got there earlier the next part may never have happened.

That is not me blaming anyone else, all parties were in the wrong that night. We continued to make our way back home but, in the distance, we saw 3 of the lads that had tried to attack us. They were at a petrol station and looked to be washing their hands and weapons at the machine that you use to fill up your washer bottle in your car.

They hadn't seen us, this is the moment I wish the police were there or some force would grip me and say this was not a good idea, but no at the time we were angry that they had tried to seriously injure us and we wanted revenge.

We split up and ambushed the lads as they left the garage. It makes me sick to my stomach now, but we absolutely went to town on these lads until all were out cold lying motionless on the ground. I thought, we have just murdered these lads.

By this time, we know now that the local CCTV operator was guiding the police to our locations. Couple of minutes later we were arrested and slung into the back of a police van and taken to Reading police station.

We were stripped of our boots and clothes and placed in separate cells until we were sober enough for interview.

Sat in my cell I was fearing the worst, I thought we had just killed 3 lads and I would now spend the rest of my life in prison. I was so frightened, and it was all the unknown, what will happen, will I see my family again. A million thoughts rushed around my head and I had time to run scenario after scenario around to see what outcome I could put together. Sitting in this tiny piss stinking cell looking at a shiny metal toilet was a wakeup call.

That morning we had interviews under caution as I did previously and unbelievably, the duty solicitor recommended me to give "no comment" replies under questioning. I did as I was told but I didn't feel comfortable and always wanted to speak the truth, so I did. They told me that the lads we had fought with were pretty banged up, at the time I wasn't that bothered about them, other than they were alive and going to make it, thankfully they did.

I said earlier that these were two of the worst years of my life, not only did I let myself down, I let my family down, the Regiment down and in doing so tarnished the good work I did in

Iraq and now I felt no better than a druggy claiming benefits. I was low, we pulled together and from the 5 of us who were arrested and charged, 3 of us took the full wrap. There was sketchy cctv footage and it painted us in a bad light, clearly looked like an ambush in the street. Holding our hands up we were in the wrong and awaited our punishments.

Not only did I have 1 violent conviction, I was facing yet another, we were bailed to appear at Basingstoke magistrates court for what we thought was our punishment outcome.

We all stood and confirmed our names in the dock; however, the proceedings were brought to a very swift close. We were looking at a charge of Affray which in a nutshell, is starting a riot. The magistrate said that the Magistrates court was not the place to deal with such an alleged crime and instead it should be heard at Crown Court instead.

This shit just got real; we were advised that there was real potential for us to be given a lengthy prison sentence for our actions. From being trained killers to quivering wrecks we all thought that this would be our careers and lives over.

Facing a lengthy wait for a court date, we finally arrived at Winchester Crown court in the June 2005. Supported by our regimental officers, we were all dressed in our military number 2 dress, green trousers and tunic, silver buttons, Iraq campaign medal on the left side of our chests, maroon beret and parachute wings on our arms.

We were told to bring a small wash kit with us, in case the inevitable were to happen.

We were all 3 of us stood in a sealed off dock this time, there was a long wooden bench I could feel behind my knees, glass screen in front of us and directly opposite us was the jury and the "victims" of our attack.

If we had not of defended ourselves that night and they stabbed us to death it would have been very different. The Law however was the Law and we were deemed to be the aggressive party with the end result of someone else getting hurt. I will be brutally honest when it came to be causing these men harm, it was far to easy for us to do. This takes me back to our training, physically and mentally, toughened through hard training and brainwashed you may say to some degree. We were taught to attack without remorse but then be controlled, we were not this time, beer and the willingness not to let anything happen to each other took over.

We all 3 pleaded guilty as charged for Affray, we waited to hear our fate, there was something in our defence that may stop us from going to prison.

One of our officers stood up in front of the court to give the judge and jury some background of us, he said that we stood fast against a foreign enemy in Iraq and we all had performed our duties as soldiers with the upmost professionalism and integrity throughout our short careers so far and up held the British Army's core values of courage, discipline, respect for others, integrity, loyalty and selfless commitment, whilst in uniform. He went on to say that this was the only time we had let ourselves down and that we had brought our Regiment into disrepute. However, with current tensions in Afghanistan brewing, we will need these outstanding soldiers to defend our country once more, so please could the court and jury take this into account.

I was so grateful for the support this officer had shown us, it was our fault and our fault alone as to why we were stood in the dock that day but we all wanted to put it right.

The court was adjourned whilst the jury could make a decision and the judge can consider his punishment for us.

Then came our shit sandwich as we called it in the trade, which is normally shit news, followed by better news, followed by shit news.

The judge spoke and expressed his disappointment in us professional soldiers, "who should know better" he went on to say that with the skills we had been taught, we were in fact, lethal weapons and the outcomes of the men's injuries could have been far worse. Good news for us in the middle of the shit sandwich was that "thanks to your officers statement and a pending operational deployment to Afghanistan, I am not going to send you to prison, instead I am going to hit you where it hurts, in your pockets!" relief I felt for a brief second, I am not going to prison. The last bit of the shit sandwich was this. "instead of a prison sentence I am going to make you pay £3000 pounds each to the victims as damages and give you all a 12-month suspended prison sentence.

Bollocks that was a blow and half, money was our lifeline, no more beer for us for the next few months. The suspended sentence part meant that if we were to commit another offence within 12 months it was going to be route direct to jail, do not pass go and definitely do not collect £200.

Thankfully back in 2005 was my last conviction and to date now nearly in 2021 I am glad to say that I have become a better person, I will go into the reasons for this a little later on.

Just my advice to you is try if you can to stay out of trouble with the police, once you get these types of convictions, I am afraid they never go away, every single job I apply for, be that as a Paramedic later on, or a kids Rugby coach, I have to explain why I have these convictions, how I have reformed and why I would not do anything like that again. It is just a constant reminder and although I have done my time and paid the price it does not look good when a new employer sees these convictions.

Lets be honest though, it was not theft, messing with kids, fraud or anything else, it was 2 punch ups that ended up with someone being hurt, I am not trying to make light of it I am just saying had it been one of the above mentioned I would have never been able to gain meaningful employment.

Although I am not proud of these convictions, honesty and understanding employers have never turned me down and have always put their faith in me to do the right things, we all fuck up and get knocked down, but we pick ourselves up and push on, if only it was as easy as that.

CHAPTER 18

Afghanistan looming

I will start this chapter by giving you a little taste of what it was like in Afghanistan during our 6-month deployment in 2006, then take you back to the build-up and key actions which I was involved in.

The following is from Brigadier Ed Butler CBE DSO, Commander UK Task Force Helmand on his time in charge and will give you a bit of an idea of what is to come.

My six months as commander British Forces Afghanistan, in 2006, was the most challenging and risk intensive command tour I have undertaken in my career. Over the six bloody and ferocious months in Helmand Province the 3 PARA Battlegroup was involved in some 500 contacts, with half a million rounds of small arms and over 13,000 artillery and mortar rounds being fired. It saw the blooding of the Apache attack helicopter and the joint Helicopter Force flying over 100 CASEVAC (Casualty Evacuation, often by helicopter) missions to extract some 170 casualties- with sadly 33 KIA (Killed in Action). Contacts could last for six-eight hours, with Paratroopers fighting in 50 degrees centigrade and carrying 70lb of equipment 'fighting order'. Young men quickly matured beyond their years; battle hardened by an intensity not witnessed since the Korean War. Some would spend weeks fighting and sleeping in their body armour and helmets, often snatching no more than a few minutes rest be-

tween enemy attacks and drinking water the temperature of a decent brew. Phenomenal stuff.

Hundreds of Taleban were killed and injured, but not once was I in any doubt that the Battle group was in danger of being defeated. By the end of the summer the Taleban had been tactically beaten, deciding to take on members of 16 Air Assault Brigade in a conventional and attritional fight. In my judgement the Taleban seriously underestimated the professionalism, raw courage, and self-belief of the Airborne Soldier; the current wearers of the maroon beret more than live up to the reputation of their forefathers.

The cost of this break-in battle into southern Afghanistan was high in blood and treasure and we will never forget those brave men who paid the ultimate sacrifice, including Corporal Bryan Budd VC and Corporal Mark Wright GC, daring all to win all. All their names, along with the towns of Now Zad, Musa Qaleh, Sangin and Gereshk will remain firmly listed in regimental history. And rightly so.

I salute the courage and endeavours of all those who I was privileged to lead across the UK task force, 16 Air Assault Brigade and especially those in the 3 PARA Battle Group. (Brigadier Ed Butler CBE DSO).

There you go, Afghanistan wrapped up. If only. Afghanistan as you probably know had been at war for decades and since the departure of the Russians in 1988, the whole of Afghanistan but namely Helmand Province had become a real lawless state and warlords across the country fought to retain all the spoils but resulted in the Mujahedeen factions seizing power of the area.

In 1999 peace talks in the country broke down and with the uprising of the Taleban, they now were fighting with the country's war lords for power. The US imposed trade sanctions on the Taleban in July 1999 and threatened military action on them. Fighting spread from north to south, into Helmand and at this time training camps were popping up to train Al Qaeda fighters who had arrived from the middle east and pledged their allegiance to the lunatic that was known as Osama Bin Laden.

On 11th September 2001 remember I told you I was in training at the AFC Harrogate, this was pivotal and the main reason that we did end up deploying to Helmand. 16 Air assault Brigade were deployed to Afghanistan in November 2001, and within a few short months it was declared that the Taleban were defeated in the capital, Kabul and it was tea and medals all round. The lads who were on that tour said it was buckshee and very little went on.

The strap line we were told was that we as a Battle Group would be going out to southern Afghanistan to provide security and stability to the area to allow the delivery of reconstruction. What a load of bollocks that was to start with. In my opinion it was to stop the Taleban supply lines of heroin to the west. Opium poppy trade in Helmand was rife, and the only viable source of income, so in my mind, we went to Iraq for oil and afghan for drugs, but that's just me.

CHAPTER 19

<u>Preparation and Oman</u>

In August 2005 we were given the official warning order to prepare for potential operations in Afghanistan although no official government statement had yet been released. How would we prepare for peace support missions? I tell you how, as Airborne soldiers of the 3 PARA Battlegroup, we would prepare as always for all eventualities, we all knew how robust the Taleban were and even if the intelligence suggests there were minimal Taleban in the area, there was always a chance of them showing up for the party when the paras are in town.

As usual we started our preparation for Afghanistan and the 50 degrees heat in a place called Otterburn, Northumberland, where it was normally minus 5, makes you smile really but always goes back to that saying: train hard, fight easy.

The training in Otterburn was not peace support role focused at all. As normal we as the small FST were embedded with the infantry companies, and this time I was to serve alongside A company 3 PARA. This is where we met some of the mortar lads, cracking but slightly weird blokes. We welcomed Guy Roberts and Mark Wright to the team. With those 2 additional lads, we not only had the capability to deliver artillery on top of the enemy, but now mortars too, maximum firepower for such a small team which would be a vital part of the Infantry company.

We completed a range of different training drills, which included an air assault phase where we would rapidly deploy by helicopter and push straight into different scenarios, things like Fighting in Built Up Areas (FIBUA) concentrating on tactics and manoeuvres. We conducted live fire training, using our personal weapon systems alongside live artillery and mortar firing in support of the infantry attacks. It was physically demanding; however, it would be the closest thing we could do in preparation for what was to come.

In January 2006 we were rounding off our final training package, alongside Estonian and Danish allies. This was brilliant to finish our in-country build up training. During the final attacks we deployed as a battlegroup by Parachute, in one of the largest peacetime drops since WW2. As normal there was rumour that we were all going to parachute into Afghanistan, as a show of force. This sounded amazing and exciting however knowing what I know now and the dangers that lurked out there, I for one am bloody glad we did not lob in.

On the same day that we were sat back-to-back at RAF Brize Norton, fully kitted and ready to parachute onto Everleigh drop zone (DZ), primed to attack Copehill Down training village, the official announcement from Government came. The UK Task Force was given the green light to deploy on a 'peace support mission' to Helmand Province, Afghanistan.

We were of course not told of this announcement until the end of the attack following the best words any soldier can wish to hear, "endex, endex" music to our ears, that was the end of the exercise and we had been validated and approved as a battlegroup to go anywhere in the world for any type of mission needed at the time.

We were not the brightest bunch of blokes granted; however, alarm bells rang when we had just completed the hardest training package we had all done before in preparation for a peace support mission. I do not think we were told the whole story.

No disrespect at all to any other Units or Brigades but if we were headed to southern Afghanistan, where no British Soldiers had been before, to a place that had been at war for centuries, the government obviously wanted to send the best, in my opinion 3 PARA Battlegroup was this.

Just to give you a brief overview of the Battle Group and what it consists of. The lead infantry Battalion at the time was the 3rd Battalion, The Parachute Regiment. They were supported by elements of 16 Air Assault Brigade who all had the same capability as the infantry to deploy by air assault or parachute. There was us as the airborne artillery, 7th Parachute Regiment, RHA. There was the Medic element who would look after us all should the worst happen, 16 Close Support Medical Regiment. The Sappers from 51 Parachute Squadron. The 156 Provost Company, Royal Military Police, 8 Close Support Troop, 7th Battalion Royal Electrical Mechanical Engineers (REME), 13 Air Assault Regiment Royal Logistics Corp (RLC). Along with these special units we had the Brigades elite Pathfinder Platoon and Apache attack helicopters from 3 Army Air Corp. Without all these specialist units, one could not operate independently. We all came through the same type of training, P Company and had each other's backs, no matter what.

As the title of this chapter suggests, we were to deploy one more place before Afghanistan in a final preparation package. We were deployed to Oman which is a country on the southeastern coast of the Arabian Peninsula, western Asia and a little fact is the oldest independent state in the Arab World. We would deploy to Oman to continue our training on exercise Desert Eagle, catchy title hey? Where we would get a taste of the environment we would likely be operating in in Afghanistan. We were to be based in a camp in the middle of the desert for 6 weeks.

The reason for this deployment as mentioned above was 2 fold, yes it would give us some acclimatisation training in the heat and the dust of the desert, but the main reason was to train alongside the new additions to the brigade, the Apache attack helicopter. What a piece of kit, it would be the first time in British Military history that the Apache helicopters would be used, first in Oman, then later on in Afghanistan, they would turn out to be a real life saving piece of equipment.

Unfortunately, I cannot go into all the specifics of the aircraft, but what I will tell you is that the training in Oman would be fantastic. Firstly, as a group we were allowed to speak with the pilots of 3 Army Air Corp and have some great dialogue on who can do what for whom.

Not only was the Apache a standoff surveillance asset it was also a close combat attack helicopter. With its amazing fire-power coming from a 30mm cannon controlled by the pilot's helmet, it had an array of other missiles that could target the enemy with pinpoint precision if needed. The benefits of the training with Apaches meant that anyone of any rank of the ground, would have the capability to conduct a Close Combat Attack (CCA) mission with ease; from the most junior private soldier to a Brigadier, it was simple to do and in Afghanistan later on it would prove invaluable.

We trained and we trained with these fantastic aircraft and now in my team I had a Forward Observation Officer, Matt Armstrong, aka Lego head, his assistant, Taff Seaward, myself as the signaller/ operator, Mark Wright and Guy Roberts as the Mortar Fire Controllers (MFC). This was the best Military Team I had ever been in, Matt Armstrong who was a Captain was such a fantastic leader and role model and whom to this day I try to base my style on. Taff Seaward, as you can tell, is welsh unfortunately, but one of the best blokes around, highly experienced, fit and motivated. And the two mortar lads what can I say? Mark Wright who was really professional and quiet until he needs to shout! He was a real team player and very Scottish! We were leading in the home nations representation in our group, then there was Guy Roberts aka Posh PARA, with a name like Guy, he had to be posh right? What a great bunch of men and it was a pleasure to be in the team with them.

The training paid off and we were slick and effective as a team, got to know each other on a personal level, swap stories and bonded. Once again it was not all work out in Oman and we did get some time to go to the beach, yes, the beach in a lovely place called Salalah! It was truly welcomed and such a beautiful place. No beer unfortunately, however this didn't spoil our fun, we jumped in the Arabian Sea, chilled out on the sand with the sun on our faces and drew massive cocks in the sand as you would expect from British Soldiers on tour.

It felt brilliant and it was part of that work hard, play hard mentality and all of us at that stage needed a break. We would chat about Afghanistan and what we thought it would be like. Do you think we will lose blokes? Would the Taleban want to fight? We were talking ourselves up and giving it the big one, but do not forget in Iraq we never really got to take on our enemy on a personal level and it was all from afar. There were elements of excitement about going to Afghanistan but for me some reservations, as I knew their history.

One finally jolly before we headed back to the UK.

CHAPTER 20

Battle of Mirbat

On the 19th July 1972 during the Dhofar Rebellion which was supported by communist guerrillas saw the Battle of Mirbat. Why am I telling you this? Well, we had the opportunity to visit the site of the battle and it was a real eye opener and chilling experience all together. At the time back in 1972, nine members of the Special Air Service (SAS) where in the area training local soldiers and to compete against the Popular Front for the Liberation of the Occupied Arabian Gulf (PFLOAG) guerrillas for the 'hearts and minds' of the Omani people.

The SAS where based in a building called the British Army Training Team (BATT) house near the port of Mirbat.

At 6 am the BATT house was attacked by the PFLOAG or Adoo as the locals called them. Members of the SAS ran to the top of the building and assessed what was going on. This situation the SAS found themselves in will be nearly mirror image of our predicament in Sangin Afghanistan later.

There was no order in the beginning to return fire from the officer in charge Mike Kealy, as he thought it was the friendly Omani Army returning from a night picket duty.

Mike Kealy soon realised that the friendlies around his position had all been killed, the order was given to all members of the SAS to open fire and defend the BATT house.

Back in the day they used L1 A1 self-loading Rifles (SLR), this weapon system as a 7.62 calibre round, and if it hits you, you're dead.

The Adoo were aware of the range of the SAS weapons and although they suffered a few casualties, the fire power from the top of the BATT house was not enough,

At this point there were 9 men from the SAS and a hand-full of Omani intelligence officers facing an onslaught from around 200–300 Adoo guerrillas - not great odds.

The bravery now shown by Sgt Talaiasi Labalaba to run through the enemy incoming fire to a nearby 25lb Howitzer, artillery piece was nothing short of amazing. He managed to single handily operate this weapon against the incoming Adoo, normally it would take a team of up to 6 people to operate it. This took the pressure away from the BATT house, but unfortunately after near point-blank firing of the 25lb Gun he was fatally shot and was killed in action (KIA). For his actions during the battle, he was awarded a mention in dispatches.

Another 2 troopers ran to his aid but unfortunately, they were too late, Tommy Tobin and Sekonaia Takavesi were both hit. Sekonaia was not fatally wounded but Tobin took a round to his face and was also KIA.

Fortunately, if I can say that communications were established with the Royal Omani Air Force and airstrikes were called in to neutralise the threat, had this not have happened, the battle would have certainly been lost.

Why would I give you this story? Well, later on there are some similarities in what we faced in Afghanistan, but the main reason is to let you know how I felt when I visited this place. We arrived at the site of this amazing, historic battle where 9 Men of the SAS fought off up to 300 Adoo, and the hairs were up on the back of my neck. I remember it being so quiet and peaceful, it was now a little fishing port. The terrain had not changed, the BATT house was still standing and the gun pit where Laba was taking on the enemy was still there.

We were walking in the footsteps of some of the bravest men there had been, it was a beautiful day, sunny and hot and no wind to whip up the dust. There were a few kids playing around the BATT house and on the beach. It was so peaceful. It was hard to put myself in the SAS shoes, yes we could imagine where they were stood and what terrain they faced, but could not fully comprehend the noise, confusion and sheer terror that they faced on this day of days.

The most surreal thing for me was that, everything had been left after the battle, you could see bullet holes in and around the outside structure of the BATT house, there were bullet casings littered over the whole area and even scorch marks and holes where the Omani Airforce had dropped bombs on to the advancing Adoo.

We discussed between us, where we would have stood and how we would have defended the area and it was easy, as we had not had to deal with such an incident. Could we have done what these brave men did? I would like to think so but again, who would know until we had felt what it was like to be involved in such a kinetic action.

I felt truly humbled to have this chance to visit such an historic place, where fellow British Soldiers had fought so bravely and made the ultimate sacrifice. It was an amazing experience and one I shall forever treasure.

Our training in Oman came to an end, we were fitter, had a great team, and felt really well prepared for what was to come, whatever that may be.

We flew back to the UK and was granted one week leave before we had to return to Colchester, our new home and prepare to depart once again abroad, this time to Helmand Province, Southern Afghanistan on a peace support mission.

We were in for a quite different mission than advertised.

CHAPTER 21

The Briefing

We arrived back from leave a little apprehensive with our deployment to Afghanistan. Goodbyes to our families never got any easier and as from my mum's previous statement, they put on a brave face for me but they were falling apart inside. I still cannot imagine how much hurt they went through with me in Iraq and now Afghanistan, it was heart-breaking for them.

It was great to see all the lads back from leave safe and sound, there was never a question of anyone going absent without leave, AWOL due to the very real fear of not wanting to let their mates down. We were going to Afghanistan and none of us had a clue what we were about to face, although with our pre-deployment brief, someone obviously knew what it would be like.

I cannot remember who took the briefing but figure it must have been Intelligence Corp or similar. We all paraded and got sat down in the gym and waited for our brief. Not ready for what I was about to hear, I was sat next to my best bud Babs and a few others, we were chatting shite between ourselves until we were told to 'shut the fuck up' from our Battery Sergeant Major (BSM).

The briefing commenced; we were all sat in a hollow square looking at a screen with some photos on. The Ariel photos were of Camp Bastion, our home although brief for the deployment.

All you could see on the pics was some shabby tents, hesco bastion (tall sandbags with cages) and sand, what a shithole we thought.

Briefing was rolling on into a few different bits and bobs, we were nodding away until the presenter said,

"Blokes are going to die out here, I shit you not".

We were not ready to hear this, nor had we ever heard such a statement before. I said to Babs:

"We went to war in Iraq and they never said that to us? Do they know something that we don't"?

We were all back in the room now at this point, listening to every word. Intelligence from our reconnaissance mission, saw that the Taleban were flooding into Helmand from Pakistan and will be ready to hit you when you land. Peace support mission?! I am thinking to myself; this was a scary prospect. If were not all worried at this point, the captain presenting then said another belting thing,

"Look around gents, people in this room will not return home from Afghanistan, look after each other and prepare you families".

I could not believe what this lunatic was saying to us, prepare your families! 'sorry Mum, Dad got to tell you that I may not be back from Afghan and this Int Corp officer told us to let you know!!' imagine this? In my head I was not going to die and neither were my mates, deploy, smash some Taleban and get home, if only it was this easy and if only it happened. I am afraid to say that the Int Corp officer, was right and predictions later on unfortunately became a very real reality.

CHAPTER 22

<u>Helmand Province</u>

As before we checked into RAF Brize Norton ready for our 5-star treatment with RAF airlines to our final destination Southern Afghanistan, Helmand Province. If memory serves me correctly, we flew out in early April 2006. Our first port of call was Kabul, the capital city of Afghanistan. We landed in darkness, with helmets on, and body armour strapped tight to our chests and braced ourselves for a very short and sharp arrival on the ground. No lights at all in the cabin and nor from the outside. Stale air went through the cabin as around 300 Paratroopers, who had probably had a curry the night before, it was stinking. We hit the deck with a thud, and that was us in the country.

At this point we were on our own, no mobile phones, no pictures or letters from loved ones, everything was stripped from our possession. The only things we had to identify us at this point were our dog tags, which had our surname, initial, service number and blood group, that was it.

Without much time to get a feel for where we were, we got hold of our kit, loaded onto a Hercules C130 transport plane, and set off for, Kandahar, where the Americans were already set up. From there on to Camp Bastion, where we would remain until we were deployed forward on deliberate operations.

In early April, the camp was just a shell, with running water only on for a couple hours a day, constant power cuts and catering based on field rations. Day by day, Bastion seemed to grow, sewers would be dug, new tents would pop up daily and by the start of May there were nearly 2000 British Troops together as one. We now had a fighting force which included, 3 Para, 7 Para RHA, 51 Para Squadron, 16 CS Med Regiment and 9 Regiment Army Air Corp.

The next couple of weeks, we were prepping for operations, we test fired our weapon systems, received daily briefings, and helped orientate new arrivals into camp. As we did in Iraq, we made sure our wills were signed and dated, and we all spent some quiet time, writing a letter to our parents or loved ones, just in case we got the good news on tour. Not all the boys did this, some felt superstitious about it and did not want to risk it. For me I always decided to write one which I kept on my person, it said.........

Mom, Dad if this letter has gotten to you, I am really sorry. I know I have put you through the mill in the past and for that I am sorry. I know you will be hurting right now, but I don't want you to blame yourselves or anyone else, it was my decision to go and I wouldn't have changed it for the world. You are the best Mum and Dad in the world, and I love you very much. I hope in the end I did you proud. Tell Drew I love him and give everyone my best, celebrate the good times and do not dwell on this, I was here with my mates and I know they will look after me here and you back at home. Love you Dave.

At the time I wrote this it felt like I could crack on now, with freedom and do the job I trained for. I wrote 2 copies of this letter, one I kept with me and one I left back in Bastion just in case I was blown up and everything was destroyed. To this day my mum and dad never new I wrote these letters and glad that they never had to read them, I wish this was the case for all who deployed, sadly it was not.

First action, our team got the nod that we would be going on the first operation of the tour. Matt Armstrong our boss told me and Taff to get our shit squared away as we would be deploying forward with A Company 3 Para. I was buzzing, the first deployment and the chance to get out on the ground. The boss went away on a briefing and me and Taff got our kit ready. We were extremely nervous, apprehensive and a little excited but were none the wiser if we would be going on a deliberate op or a peace support one.

Matt returned and we went to his tent for a briefing. Excitement building and the nerves in the pit of my stomach we awaited his brief, it started with, "Sorry Benny, you're not coming on this one".

After hearing this, I felt as flat as a pancake,

"What do you mean I'm not coming boss?!"

"There is limited room on the helos (helicopters) and me and Taff will just be going on this one".

I was gutted and felt like I had been kicked out the team. You should always be careful what you wish for, granted, I just wanted to get out there with my mates and do the job.

He went on to brief us and the mission was to mount a cordon and search a walled compound just to the east of Now Zad. The company would fly in 4

Chinook helicopters and land to the north and south of the target, as to secure the area as soon as possible. The building was supposed to be a weapons factory. The company would be supported by 2 Apache helicopters after they got on the ground.

I am missing a chance to shoot the baddies here, but orders were orders and that was that. Team effort as always, I helped the lads prepare their kit and wished them well for a safe and successful mission.

Me and a few of the lads went up to the helipad to watch all the guys leave, we were gutted. Selfishly I wanted them to get out to the location, find nothing and get back, I wanted it to be uneventful for them so there was no story for them to tell, but of course the main one was to get them back in one piece.

The op was under way the company landed on around 12 midday. 3 Chinooks landed safely and the OC (Officer Commanding) and his tactical group remained airborne in a command and control aspect.

As soon as the lads landed the Taleban opened fire on them, no messing this is our country, and we want you out. The lads had never experienced such ferocity of attacks but bravely fought back to defend themselves.

Thankfully, the Taleban incoming fire went over the heads of our boys and they could manoeuvre safely into position.

During this contact it was the first time in British history that the Apache attack helicopter was used in battle. The Apaches were engaging and destroying Taleban in the area, this was confirmed by the lads on the ground who had to fight through them to get into the vicinity of the target location. Taff said later that the fire coming in from the Apaches was pinpoint accurate and within remarkably close proximity to our own troops.

During the attack, some intelligence came in that a Taleban leader was in and around the building, so the company pushed through the attack to try and apprehend him. Taff and Matt pushed forward with the lead section to sweep the area, they identified Taleban firing points and Matt directed an A10 American Tank Buster into action in an attempt to neutralise the firing point, which they managed to do.

The firefight continued and the company was ordered to withdraw to the inner cordon, Taff explained that he saw Taleban ferociously running towards the company and he, along with others, had to engage them with small arms fire. What a feeling this must have been for him!

There were numerous Taleban confirmed killed and unfortunately there was a civilian caught in the crossfire. He was treated by the company medic and Casevac to Bastion for treatment. The Taleban kept pushing on towards the cordon and a two man Rocket Propelled Grenade Team (RPG) were identified and swiftly dealt with.

Thankfully, there were no injuries from this op and all the company assets returned to Bastion to tell the tale.

As you could probably tell, I was not best happy, I was so glad to see Matt and Taff return, of course I was, Taff was buzzing and had an influx of adrenaline going. He got to meet the Taleban, engage them and take them out. Matt and Taff had been shot at which none of us had ever been, and the best part, they survived to tell the tale. I would later find out for myself how it felt but you could say that it is better than any drug, when you are dishing it out but when it comes to taking it back, it is a very different story.

It was a successful first mission, everyone came back safe, several Taleban were confirmed killed and the Apaches had proved to be a massive asset.

So much for the peace support mission.

CHAPTER 23

First into Kajaki

After all the build-up training with Matt, Taff, Mark, and the rest of the team, I was side-lined, or at least that is how it felt. It was clear that from now on, all the direct operations would need split teams, this was due to the number of aircraft we had in theatre. The fact was there was not enough and by August 2006, our forces would be spread so thinly across Helmand it was going to cause issues.

My time did eventually come, and I was briefed that I would be going to a place called Kajaki, it sounded ok. apparently, there was not much going on and it will be a bit of a jolly for me, so I was told. I will be honest, I wanted to be on the ground at that stage engaging the Taleban. Once again, be careful what you wish for.

I was to deploy to Kajaki with a fantastic small team, Karl Brennan, Charlie Aggrey, Martin Lewis who I knew well from my Regiment. They were a fantastic bunch and if nothing else, I know I would be looked after, they were all seniors with so much experience, so it made me feel better about the next part. We were told that we also had another 2 lads going with us, Andy Reid, who was a Medic from 16 CS Regiment and Swifty who was a Coldstream guard, randomly.

It was our task to deploy to Kajaki and defend the area. The worrying news was that we would not be going alone, we would deploy alongside a Platoon of Afghan National Army Soldiers who we knew nothing about, and potentially could turn on us at any minute.

We were also told there would be an American who we would make contact with on the ground and bring us up to speed on things in the area.

As normal we received very sketchy details about what the hell, we would be getting ourselves into.

Kajaki itself was at the top of the Sangin valley. It was home to a hydro-electric power plant that was built somewhere between 1955-1975 and was financed by the Republic of Afghanistan and the Americans. They however abandoned this project when the Soviet Army invaded the country.

This was another important area that needed defending as there were plans to replace the turbine in the plant which would then provide much needed electric to Southern Afghanistan.

We packed out kit and jumped on the Chinook Helicopters at Bastion and made our way at low level through the valley to Kajaki, I had not seen anything but sand to this point, but we were in for a very welcome surprise.

Flying over compounds and turning sharply round every bend I caught site of a mint blue river which looked massively out of place in this War-torn country.

The noise of the rotors and the fragrant smell of Jet A1 fuel engulfed the cabin. Looking across to the lads, they looked relaxed and not really concerned about anything, they were old-school compared to me and it made me relax knowing that I was with them. I could see the Kajaki Dam now which looked so inviting along with the surrounding mountains, what a beautiful place and to this day I always comment that it is one of the most beautiful places I had ever seen.

We banked hard to the left and touched down on the Helicopter Landing Site (HLS), ramp opened, and the loadmaster gave us the thumbs up to run off the back. We threw one strap of our

Bergan's over our shoulder and ran off the back of the aircraft and felt a warm blast of the two jet engines, then the continued heat of Kajaki itself. We were the first British troops on the ground in Kajaki, ever, no one can ever take that fact away. It is normal procedure when entering a hot zone to form a defensive position so that we could be ready to return fire to enemy should they engage us as soon as the aircraft left.

We did this, down on our belt buckles and waited for the chinook to leave. With a big downwash from the rotors it lifted and buggered off back to Bastion.

"Welcome to Kajaki, mother fuckers" was the cry from a tubby bloke in the distance.

We were thinking who they hell is this, John Wayne? Not John Wayne but Kajaki John, what a legend. To this day none of us had a clue who he worked for. CIA? FBI? Not a clue!

He was a short tubby bloke, who wore chinos and a waistcoat that carried god only knows what. He has an AK47 in his possession and a pistol on his hip, short grey hair with a really dodgy moustache but one of the best handshakes in the business. He gave us the tour.

The Kajaki compound consisted of brick buildings at the base of some high ground, had the look and the feel of a military training camp. There was a swimming pool, full of green shitty water and 2 gates, north and south. The southern gate gave you access to the local town of Tangay, the northern gate gave us access to the high ground from where we would operate from.

For the first few weeks there was nothing going on in Kajaki, we swam in the reservoir, we fished, and we jumped from a tower into the stunning fresh water of the dam. We observed daily from the highest peak that was named Sparrow Hawk, it was a testing climb every day, but we loved it up there. We felt safer up in the hills as it was a perfect vantage point. Down in the lower compound it was secured by the Afghan National Army and some local contractors who were dodgy as. Kajaki John told us to never take our weapons off them and be prepared to drop them if they become hostile as they could be Taleban informants. John had massive balls, before our arrival he was there on his own. I asked him what he would do if it kicked off.

He said, "Come here I will show you".

He took me to a little lock up down the bottom of the lower compound, he opened the door and there was a rucksack hanging off a hook. It was his Escape and Evasion bag and held, sophisticated radio equipment, rations and water. He was some Rambo bad ass for sure.

I got nervous every time John was around the local contractors as he was fairly aggressive to them and there was even a couple of times where he drew his pistol and pointed it right at them. It got very tense at times and we spoke about John as a team and thought up an action plan if it ever kicked off. We would have to take the lot of them out, probably John included, as he was always in their faces. He knew what he was doing and was obviously an experienced operator. Very secretive, he would tell us not to go around certain areas at certain times and you would see a Black Hawk American helicopter land now and then to resupply him.

A few weeks in, we built up a routine and a pattern of life in the area, clearly someone had tipped the Taleban off that we were there and gave them the information that we were spread thinly on the ground.

We started to receive incoming Taleban mortars, with accuracy, they would drop them in the lower compound and even on top of the hill we were observing from. Thankfully, no one was hurt during these bombardments, but it frightened me to death. We could see the firing point, there would be a flash but then it would be pure luck where the shell would land. We would count from the flash until impact and take cover as best we could. Seconds before impacting you would here the woooosh then the explosion of the shell. We had a little bit of this in Iraq but this time the fire was more accurate and at a sustained rate of fire. We would receive 10-12 rounds every attack for days on end and some landed as close as 20 metres away from us which was scary. Thankfully, we had defensive positions set but there was nothing we could do to defend these attacks.

The reason for this was that we had no artillery or mortar support at this stage, our personal weapons would not reach the enemy, and the only thing we had to combat against the threat was Charlie. He was a JTAC (Joint Tactical Air Controller) and he would use his skills to request friend's aircraft to engage the enemy. The trouble was, we never knew when they would attack and by the time we had an aircraft they would have gone, it was a frustrating period as they were getting the upper hand.

Every day we would receive intelligence via our ANA counterparts that they could hear the Taleban saying that they were a thousand strong and were going to attack us. They clearly knew we were spread thinly, and the reality was that if the Taleban did try to have a go, they would have very easily succeeded.

What we had to do as a Team was ridiculous. In an attempt to draw the Taleban into a fight and make them believe that there were more of us than there was we all split up across the high ground. once we were given a signal, we would all start to fire into different locations where we had previously been attacked from. We only had personal weapons, all the lads had SA80's and I had a 5.56 Light Machine Gun. We filled our magazines with tracer rounds and just before last light we would give it some!

Between us all we put 100s of rounds down into those pre-recorded areas purely for affect, we could not see the enemy, but we had to do something to deter them else we would have been overrun.

It was ridiculous but it worked, the attacks became fewer and fewer and the intelligence suggested that the underestimated our numbers. I spent around a month and half in Kajaki and although some scary bum twitching moments with incoming mortars we were all ok and came through it. It could have been worse, it did get to a point where we had to plead with command to send us a General Purpose Machine Gun (GPMG) as it was the only thing that would reach the enemy should we come under attack. We did get this but clearly not enough ammunition for it and our request for Artillery or Mortar support was denied as fighting was ensuing elsewhere.

Kajaki was not a hard place to operate for me but you may be aware, following our departure and the arrival of our relief soldiers it was to be very different. As mentioned earlier my old Team consisted of Taff, Matt and Mark Wright. They were now operating in Sangin District Centre so I would not see them until the end of the Tour, however before I left Bastion I of course didn't realise that it would be the last time I ever saw Mark, as he was later deployed to Kajaki, the exact same place I had been for the last month and half and he would lose his life in a major action of the War in Afghanistan on the 6th September 2006, I will talk more about this later.

Later on, too Kajaki John as we called him would also be killed as he finally departed Kajaki in a road move and was ambushed by the Taleban, multiple ANA soldiers that I had served with in Kajaki would also lose their lives.

I returned back to Bastion from Kajaki for a brief period, as apparently, I was needed elsewhere. The first thing I heard when I arrived back was that one of our own had been KIA.

Captain Jim Phillipson of our Regiment 7th Parachute Regiment RHA. My heart sank and from all the briefings that we had; the predictions were coming true. We had been really lucky not to sustain any injuries so far, but this was to be the start of some of the bloodiest months of the tour.

Captain Phillipson, was the first British Soldier to be KIA, on the 11th June 2006 whilst out on a mobile patrol, they were engaged in a firefight with the Taleban and he was hit and killed instantly, 2 of the other lads were seriously injured whilst they attempted to treat him.

I felt quite numb and although knew this day might well happen, it has just got real, lads I know had engaged with the Taleban and this time had been injured.

A mix of emotions set in, anger, guilt, fear come rushing in at once, how would the lads have felt having to deal with this shit situation, I personally was still to find out, most of the lads had seen close combat yet I had been left out the Team, sent on a jolly to Kajaki and not really done a thing to affect the War efforts.

I was still hungry to get on the ground and fight and my time was coming.

CHAPTER 24

SANGIN District Centre

The man may leave the valley, but the valley will never leave the man (Dave Benny Bentley). I was desperate to get into the fight, get an opportunity to take on the Taleban and get some payback for the lads who had been killed. Once again, I would not be joining up with my old team, Matt, and Taff, it would be a new gang led by Jason Conway, Staff Sergeant at the time, he was a good bloke with bags of experience. I would be his assistant or ACK and we would be joined by a fresh-faced Chris Russ as signaller. From now on we would be known as, Fire Support Team 4. We also had Posh Para Robbo and Andy Carr as his number 2, along with Si Scholes.

We got together as a Team briefly before we got the call that we would be taking over as the FST at Sangin District Centre. At the time this was one of the most dangerous of places in Southern Afghanistan, along with Musa Qaleh.

The Town of Sangin, in the Helmand Valley was a notorious hot spot for the Taleban and the opium trade. The Taleban in Sangin were the judge, jury and executioner of the local population and had total control, until we arrived.

We were headed straight for the hornet's nest, to take on the Taleban in their back garden.

Once again as a team we prepped ourselves for battle in the

normal way. We were going to conduct a relief in place, (RIP) with my old Team, there would be no time to speak to each other, no handshakes or welfare checks, this would be a real in and out job into one of the most dangerous places on the planet at that time.

We made our way up to the Helipad at Camp Bastion as a team, Jase, Robbo, Andy, and Si all had vast amounts of experience as did I now, to a certain degree, but Chris who was 18 at the time had none. He had just flown out to be with us and he was green as grass; it was my job to keep him under a wing and make sure he was doing what he needed to do and importantly make sure he was kept alive and could go home after all this was over.

Chris is a lovely lad, funny but thick as mince at times, however, he would always get the job done. He is an Airborne soldier at the end of it all, as we all were so we knew that blokes left and right of us would have our backs, no matter of creed, colour, background, or unit, we are all from the same brotherhood.

The familiar sound of the Chinook's rotors starting to turn, jets cranking up and the smell of Jet A1 passing through our noses into our lungs. Nerves building and lots of questions and thoughts running through our heads. Letters to our families in our pockets and weapon systems made ready to go straight into a fight on arrival. Due to Sangin's reputation and the news that we got before we lifted made me the most frightened, I had ever been to that point. There was a fair chance that I would not be coming back from this. Taking deep breaths and looking around at the lads gave me a sense of calm, at least I was going in with these amazing blokes and if anything were to happen, I would look after them and likewise them for me.

(Sangin DC, third top window in from the right was our room)

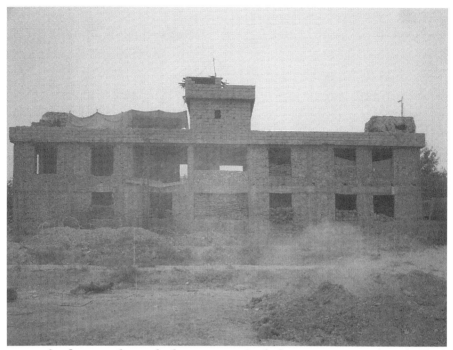

Just before we boarded, we got wind that two guys were killed at Sangin and a few injured a day ago, the seniors tried to keep it quiet, but it always gets out.

We heard that a Taleban rocket had hit the top of the building where 2 lads were sleeping, Pete Thorpe and Jabron Hashmi of the signals and intelligence corps were killed instantly, along with an Afghan interpreter, also lads were injured by the vast amounts of shrapnel that the rocket gave off. This is news that you do not want to hear before boarding a helicopter. We were all gutted, frightened, and angry. A few lads started to get mad, and you could see they wanted blood, I did too, the nerves slowly went as we lifted from Bastion on our 20-minute low level flight.

Passing over the rooftops of mud buildings we were given to two-minute out warning order and prepared to de-bus from the aircraft and allow members of A Company, who had had it so rough, to get back to Bastion in order to get their wounded treated and the bodies of Pete and Hash back safely and then onward to the UK and their families.

We come in fast and landed inside the compound attached to the District Centre, dust everywhere we could not see a thing, we all ran off the back as quickly as we could and fanned out ready for the Taleban to pounce.

I was looking around for Matt, Taff, Mark, and the rest of the boys but I could not see them. What I did see were eight blokes carrying two stretchers, with body bags on top of them, which could have only been Pete and Hash. It was a really disturbing sight and one I will never forget. God only knows how the lads felt having to deal with the rocket, the dead and injured; it must have been horrific for them, still I had not experienced this part of war, but I would not have to wait long.

Within 40-50 seconds, we were of the back of the aircraft and the dead and injured were on and en route to Bastion. Another aircraft followed and I was now safe in the knowledge that my old team were heading back for a little bit of down time at Bastion, where the risk of danger was greatly reduced.

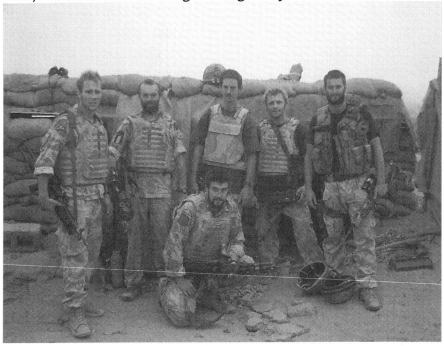

(FST 4 , left to right, Chris, Si, Guy, Andy, Jase and me front)

We were not attacked, and it was as if the Taleban knew we had dead and injured, and it seemed there was a ceasefire whilst this relief in place was conducted. You can guarantee though that this was just coincidence and the silence was due to the lads battering them the night before, following the deaths of our boys.

"Welcome to fabulous Sangin", the Company Sergeant Major said as we reached the main building in the compound.

Dusty with the odd bit of greenery around the place this used to be an Afghan police compound before we took it over. Now, surrounded by some hesco bastion, light sandbag filled walls to offer some protection. There were 2 main buildings in the complex one was completely covered and protected and the other was like a new build under construction. It was still open to the elements, with concrete pillars and posts but with extremely limited protection from incoming rockets or small arms. All the windows of the building were full of sandbags and there was evidence all-around of the contact with the Taleban, bullet holes in the walls, scorch marks in the walls and holes where rockets had previously hit.

I mentioned before there were some similarities between this place and the BATT House during the Battle of Mirbat, it had that eerie feeling about it. The lads who remained in place looked tired, dirty and all had that classic 1000-yard stare that you often see in the war movies. This, I knew was going to be the toughest time I would face, and I just wanted to make sure I did not let myself or my team down.

We were shown to our 5-star accommodation, we would be situated on the first floor of the derelict shell of a building that faced the town of Sangin. The room was concrete from floor to ceiling and approximately six metres square. It had no features, just a window overlooking the river which would play a big part of our time there later.

We dumped our kit and OCB Company gave us a briefing and orientation of the land and warned us that they had been attacked constantly whilst in Sangin and to expect imminent incoming enemy fire at any moment. Body Armour and helmets was to be worn at all times, even when sleeping, if you get a chance, he joked.

We were then led by the OC out of our room, turning left up 2 flights of concrete stairs to the infamous rooftop where most of the action had taken place. I was not prepared for what I would see next, at the top of the stairs was the room where Hash and Pete plus an interpreter had been killed only hours ago. This was our only route up and down to our FST position. This small room, all concrete again, had a big hole in it where the Taleban rocket had entered, the devastation that was left will never leave me. The bodies of the lads had obviously gone, but we could see exactly where they were positioned when the rocket hit, the smell of cordite in the air, coagulated blood everywhere up the walls, on the ceiling; bits of fabric from their clothes and broken equipment that they had obviously been carrying at the time. There was left over medical equipment which the lads would have tried desperately to use to save their lives; it was an horrendous sight which would be a constant reminder to us all every time we used the stairs. It was harrowing for us to see and we were not even there at the time. For the first time I felt that I was in a real warzone and that night the Taleban gave us a welcome.

Following our ground appreciation from the OC we were told that there were 2 main points where the Taleban liked to launch their attacks from. Looking far right from our position there was a large white building, named the Pharmacy and to our far middle distance there was a wood line, named Wombat Wood which would be the Taleban's favoured position to launch the rockets from. In between these two points there was derelict shops, a marketplace, and brick works. The thing I found slightly strange was that there was no one around, as far as the eye could see, until I experienced it for myself I could not believe that this was the most dangerous part of Afghanistan and the place with the highest amount of British fatalities to date.

There were no locals, as they had either fled the area or knew that there was a Taleban attack imminent. This indeed was the case, there was a flash of light and a whoosh followed by a loud explosion to the front of our building. Added to that was small arms fire, and the crack and thumping noise over our heads. We were under attack! We could see tracer coming from some buildings about 400 metres away from us, it was the Taleban for sure as the tracer was green in colour. It was perfectly accurate initially, very much over our heads and we all got into position on the rooftop and returned fire. "What's the firing point", "give a fucking target indication" one of the lads shouted.

The 50-calibre machine gunner next to us saw the firing point. "Watch my tracer" he yelled.

He let go with the thump of the beast of a weapon system and we all followed suit, I was firing into the area with my LMG and targeting places I thought the Taleban would be, couple of minutes went and we had the 'Seize fire' command followed by 'Watch and shoot' which meant exactly that, keep your eyes peeled and anything you're not happy with, let them have it.

The adrenaline was pumping through my veins, I was hyper-vigilant and ready to go again, I had a real feeling of exhilaration, dishing it out was fun, but taking the incoming was not. This was our first experience of a short Taleban attack, an opportunist moment and one of hundreds more to follow. I did not even see any Taleban at the time, let alone hit any, they were like ghosts.

Night fell and the temperature dropped, we had night vision available to us, along with flares and claymores set out in front of our positions. Just up the road from us in FOB Robinson were two of our 105 light Guns and my mates from I Battery, ready to support us if needed. Luckily for me, Jase and the team, Taff and Matt had already fired artillery and mortars on the majority of the positions in and around the compound and recorded them so that we could fire on them straight away should we come under attack from those positions. The lads before us had done such an amazing job and had given us the best opportunity to look after the 150 of us in the compound, it was a job that we knew had to be right or else others could be killed.

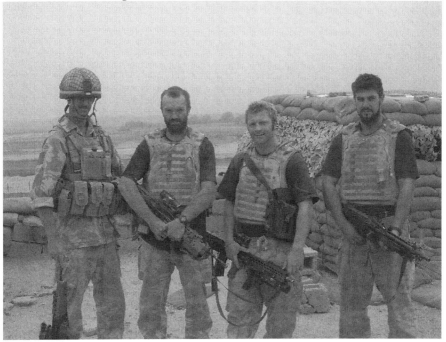

(Left to right, Guy, Si, Andy and me following a lul in the battle)

During the next few days we settled into a routine, working from the rooftops, spotting Taleban targets, and repelling their long-distance attacks. The norm was to be attacked daily by either, 107mm rockets, 7.62 AK47 rounds and Rocket Propelled Grenades (RPG) not in that order but sometimes all at once.

It was our job to locate the enemy and put something bigger and nastier on top of them. As we recorded all our targets as mentioned earlier, it was a case of making a call to the gunline.

"Hello 0 this is Delta 31 Bravo, UQ4501 3 rounds Fire for Effect, over!"

This in English meant that we wanted the two light Guns up the road in FOB Rob to fire 3 105mm high explosive shells each, onto the Target UQ4501 which this time was Wombat Wood.

We saw a flash and heard the incoming so as normal took cover, we also had some surveillance kit called MSTAR, (Man Portable, Surveillance, Target, Acquisition, Radar,) Say that after a few beers! That would give us clear evidence that there were targets in the area. Following their attacks, we would look at the radar and enemy troops would show as yellow dots on the screen. We would get the gun's reply, they would repeat back what we had sent to confirm the order and the next thing we waited for was "Shot on UQ4501 over" this meant that the Guns had fired the first rounds onto the target, we could hear in the distance the boom, boom, and the ripple overhead as they made their way to Wombat Wood. My job along with Jase was to spot where the rounds were landing and adjust them onto the target if necessary. This time there was no need, six 105mm high explosive shells set to point detonating hit the wood line with pinpoint precision. We sent our BDA, (Battle Damage Assessment) back to the gun line, morale for all, the firing stopped, and the five yellow dots on our screen were no more. The confirmation came when the intelligence officer gave us feedback from his ICOM scanner that the Taleban needed to recover their dead, this was a real boost for everyone's morale. Granted, this was not fighting in the trenches with bayonets, which was to come, it was fighting from distance, using our superior skills and weapon systems to defeat the enemy, it meant that the infantry didn't need to go out on the ground and risk being ambushed and it inflicted a big blow on the Taleban.

The Taleban were far from stupid however, and on 6th July we were waiting for resupply from two Chinook helicopters. As normal one of the platoons went out to secure the HLS in case of Taleban attacks, it was too late though. The sound of the inbound helicopters was drowned out by a Taleban ambush, we could hear the firefight ensue from the roof and could not get any information back as to where the firing point was. This meant we could not support in case of hitting our own troops. There was confusion everywhere and the lads on the ground did their best to smash the Taleban back, soon followed a radio message that no one ever wants to hear.

"Man, down man down"

A shiver went down my spine, this meant that one of the lads had been hit. I ran down to try and find out where the troops were so we could supress the enemy to assist in the casualty being withdrawn. By the time I ran down from the roof to the ops room, the lads were dragging one of the others back in. He looked alive, but the medic and his brothers from his platoon were working hard to treat his wound. Quickly he was being seen by the company doctor, but it was too late; sadly, Private Damian Jackson had been KIA aged 19. I did not know him but felt all his section's pain, it was horrific to see those lads and medical staff go to work on this young lad, who clearly knew he was going to die. I had never seen anything like this, and it caused a mix of emotions again, anger, rage, guilt, due to us not being able to help at the time. There were roughly 150 of us in Sangin and every man felt helpless. It knocked us for several days and naturally we wanted to get some pay back.

It was now time to take the fight to the Taleban, instead of waiting to be ambushed, or react to their fire, we would fight them in their back garden.

You can see Jase's footage of our time in Sangin via the BBC 3 Documentary Our War The Invisible Enemy, it will give you some context, and you get to see us naked.

CHAPTER 25

Face to Face with Terry Taleban

We knew we had to take the fight to the Taleban to maintain the upper hand in the area, so much for a peace support mission, this was proper soldiering. Jase and I would integrate with the lead sections on the ground so that if contact was made with the enemy, we could direct fires on to the targets in the knowledge that we knew where all the friendlies were. I will be honest; I was frightened to death. I knew, and had seen with my own eyes, the risks of going outside the wire, but we had a job to do. One morning under darkness I headed out with the lead platoon, we were going to set our own ambush. We set out from the District centre and patrolled up the street to the white pharmacy building, Jase, Chris, Andy and Si were on the roof providing overwatch. For the first 20 minutes, nothing happened, but clearly the Taleban were watching and waiting to attack.

I caught first sight of the infamous Taleban, we were taking a knee alongside a muddy wall and up ahead of me I saw five Taleban fighters, wearing a mix of black and white dish dash (Local dress) running cross the top of town, fully kitted out with AK47's and RPGs a plenty, clearly hurrying to get into a decent fire position. I hit my belt buckle and as I did a young Paratrooper to the side of me shouted, "contact front!" and opened fire with his GMPG, spraying a long burst of 7.62 into the group, we all then followed suit and opened up. I let three or four good bursts of 5.56 off into the path of the Taleban who were stupidly caught in no man's land. The contact was live, I gave an update to Jase and the gun line.

"Hello 0 this is Delta 31 Bravo, Contact. Wait out!"

It was fucking chaos and as the old saying goes, no plan survives contact with the enemy. Confusion ensued, I was stuck with the lead section and my old role of Artillery Observer soon went and I was part of the lead section in an infantry role. We were tasked to push forward to clear out the enemy we sighted 200 meters up the road, this bunch were not the brightest running through open ground as I said earlier, they must have been the Dad's Army of the Taleban. We took sporadic fire back but believed we had the upper hand in this fight. We made our way up the road and were given a LOE (limit of exploitation) near the pharmacy building so that we could be seen by the lads on the roof. We could here shots cracking over our heads and that was from the snipers back at the DC who had sighted Taleban in the open and dropped them where they stood. We were called to the side of the pharmacy building and the lads were still firing on a group of Taleban, but when the dust settled, it was clear that we had got them! Three dead Taleban, plus weapons. Strangely, I was buzzing with my heart pounding, feeling invincible. There were only three dead fighters though? The snipers had taken care of the others; this group of fighters were no more.

They were spread out in a wadi (a dry riverbed). One was clearly hit in the head as it was twice the size, and others it seemed in the chest and back. It was hard to tell. All dressed in robes all with full beards, their shoes and sliders were scattered around where they had fallen. It was hard to tell how old they were. They had Russian AK47 rifles with plenty of ammunition and two RPG's. A little walkie-talkie radio was found on one of them, so we took this with us.

The lads checked the bodies for traps and for intelligence. I helped the lads drag the dead Taleban around the corner to the front of the pharmacy building. We lined them up, top and tail and covered them up for dignity with some blankets that were lying around near the pharmacy and withdrew back to the DC. I had just had my first physical engagement with the enemy. What a feeling! I had previously given the orders to fire artillery onto targets, but this time it was a direct action onto a live target which in some ways felt more personal. Granted, I was not alone, which helped, but I often thought how I would feel to be in this situation, or if I were actually up to it. What would my reactions be? I was, up to it! I stood up and I honestly did not feel anything. It felt very instinctive and drill-like. You hear people say kill or be killed. There was none of that, we saw the enemy, which was a rarity and we fanned out and engaged the targets. All your training, simple fear and your reactions kick in and it was done, you do not hang around discussing whose bullet hit who. The lads had just lost Jacko, and whoever was in that area was clearly Taleban and we were proved right when recovering their weapons and equipment.

Later, on reflection I was chuffed to be part of this small action but in honesty I felt lucky that it was a direct action instigated by us and we clearly had the upper hand. It would have been hugely different had we had been ambushed or pinned down like a lot of the lads had been previously.

I felt that I had done my job well in front of the Infantry lads. For me, this was massive. They gave me kudos and we bonded further; they appreciated our role more and I have no doubt without our support there would have been many more fatalities.

This said we were now heading into 35 days with 31 of those days in contact with the Taleban. As they say, no rest for the wicked!

CHAPTER 26

Men Apart

Fighting continued day in day out for us, with only minutes in the day to catch up on some rest. The Taleban were getting smarter and more desperate in an attempt to overrun us. As it was so dangerous in the area, we were faced with a desperate situation, running low on ammunition and food. One evening I remember sitting on the rooftop with the lads and we were waiting on the RAF to parachute supplies into us. Si was on the radio chatting to them, gave them all the information they required, and we heard Fat Albert approaching. We were all quite excited at the thought of getting some supplies in for the next few weeks. The excitement wore off when the plane flew by without dropping anything, we thought they may be doing a dummy run. No. In the distance we saw three parachutes dropping from the rear of the plane about 5 km from our position, deep in Taleban territory.

"Well, we aren't fetching that then" I said.

By the time we got to those supplies they would be gone, we had just resupplied the Taleban for months, luckily it was only food and not ammunition. I must say all the lads in the team and in Sangin itself, were warriors. They fronted up to the Taleban every day and there were acts of heroism and bravery every hour of the day. An example of this bravery was Chris, our young signaller.

"Benny, I will go and get the supplies dropped, if I get killed it will only be me" he informed me.

That was from an 18-year-old boy, who is now a man, stepping up to the plate and acting selflessly for the good of others. I wish that was the case with all 18-year-olds nowadays. Chris was a fantastic bloke, who was dragged up in the Rhondda Valleys in Wales and he was now bravely serving in the Sangin Valley in Afghanistan.

Chris was at his post on the roof one day, me and a few of the lads were getting a bit of rest, cat napping away, and then the daily wakeup call - crack and thump of incoming fire. I woke up and for a few seconds wondered where the fuck I was! Dis-orientated and jabbering on, I grabbed my LMG and headed up to the roof. As I left the room, opposite me on a concrete wall was a couple of things, one was the 'wheel of fate', a cardboard cut-out with an arrow pointer that we used to spin to see what we would get that day. It had, small arms, RPG, Mortars, which to this point we had not had, and a rocket from Wombat wood, a little dark humour. On the way up the stairs, we had another sign, this time made from wood saying, Beware Two Way Range, which was highly accurate.

Once again, thinking of Pete and Hash every time we ran past where they were killed, it gave us the energy to attack. So far, we had managed to repel the daily attacks with, machine guns, ar-tillery, mortars, and cannon from a Household Cavalry Scimitar (an armoured vehicle) but when we were out on the ground, we found a whole network of Taleban tunnels that we would not be able to penetrate with the above, we needed something bigger.

With the 7.62 dirty green tracer flying in, we stayed low and managed to get to Chris.

"Where's the firing point mate? "I asked,

"Just by there," he replied,

"Where the fuck is by there, Chris?"

"Watch my tracer", he then put a burst of about 20-25 rounds of mixed 5.56 tracer into a corner of a compound 300 meters away from us.

"The cheeky bastards are getting closer "I said.

With that, we saw the muzzle flashes of the Taleban and Chris continued to engage, along with everyone else on the roof. Jase was on the radio, along with Robbo trying to get some artillery and mortars dropped in on them. A couple of minutes and the rounds came down and battered the area. This was game over for Terry Taleban, or so we thought.

"Good work Chris, you did great pal".

Ten minutes went by and all was quiet, but believe it or not, from that same position they hit us again. How on earth are they still alive? I wondered. I looked at Chris again and he was getting stuck in, but this time there was sand and debris flying up in front of him. I was thinking he was hitting the sandbag in front of the end of his gun. I ran over and kicked him up the arse,

"Watch your muzzle clearance Chris!" I shouted to him.

However, it was not him, it was Terry Taleban. That's how accurate they had become! Chris was bravely firing back without a care for his own safety and there is me thinking he is not aiming properly! What a legend he is! I would not have had anyone else in our corner.

We had to soon change tack. Clearly, by now, with the fighting worsening by the day, we needed to get the big dogs in to try and stop the Taleban in their tracks. We had Si Scholes, an absolute legend of the game, he was RAF Regiment and was our JTAC, in charge of all thing's aviation related.

With the next round of attacks in the coming weeks Si single handily pushed the Taleban back. He got our British Apache Attack Helicopters firing danger close missions in support of us on the ground. For the first time in our history, we were using American A10 Warthogs, which have a distinct whistling sound as they pass but deliver such devastating effects on the ground. They fire with a cannon on the front of the airframe and as the rounds land it is like firework night, the flashes and thumps as the rounds hit the ground was phenomenal. As soon as you see the flash you get a brrrrrrrrrrrrrrrrrup noise after it which was a great morale booster again for the troops. For the bunkers and network of tunnels he used 500 or 1000lb JDAM (Joint Direct Attack Munition) bombs from American B1 Bombers to penetrate deep into the ground. These shook the ground as they hit but were highly effective and it was clear that it started to break the will of the Taleban. Granted, it destroyed most of the town. However, it was clear that only Taleban fighters remained.

Elsewhere around Helmand, British Troops were in similar situations as us. They were also spread thinly and doing what they could. On the 1st August 2006, we had some more bad news delivered to us. One of our fellow FST officers, Captain Alex Eida from my unit, along with two others 2nd Lieutenant Ralf Johnson and Lance Corporal Ross Nicholls had all been killed whilst in contact with the enemy in Northern Helmand. They were travelling in a Sparton armoured vehicle when they were attacked with RPGs and heavy machine guns.

I knew Alex personally, he was such an amazing leader, very relaxed but enthusiastic and was one of my defending officers when I landed up in court. His guidance and wisdom for such a young man is something I will always hold on to. My thoughts at the time were with Babs and Mowgli who were on his team. They were split during the tasking and it could very well have been those lads involved. I know that thought pays a heavy toll on Babs and Mowgli and something that will forever be with them.

As we knew him so well, it caused lots of irritation and stress within my team itself. Jase was on edge. I was the same and it put a strain on Chris. It was hard to focus on the task when a fantastic man you knew had now gone forever. We did the best thing and sat down and discussed it. I did not know it at the time, but it was the best thing we did, clearing the air and getting back on track with the job in hand. The stresses of being in a firefight day in day out were starting to take its toll.

I want to pay tribute to another man who was also tragically killed whist in Sangin with us, even worse it was not through enemy action. Lance Corporal Sean Tansey of the Household

Cavalry died on the 12th August 2006 whilst conducting maintenance on his Scimitar during a lull in the fighting. He was part of that crew who were pivotal in the defence of us all in Sangin and were not shy about getting stuck in when the bullets started flying. They were an amazing bunch that I was so glad were on our side.

CHAPTER 27

<u>Bryan Budd VC</u>

It was now mid-August and the close attacks on our compound had slowed as the Taleban were getting smashed by our snipers and accurate in direct fire. A weapon system we all feared was the mortar as it could be fired from anywhere, often unseen, and land anywhere in the compound. Welcome to the party Taleban 6-man mortar Team! We started taking highly accurate mortar fire into the compound on a regular basis. This crew were no mugs and obviously were highly trained individuals. The mortars were primarily landing in the next compound along from ours, where the Royal Irish Rangers and the Engineers where based. These two units were also integral to our operations in Sangin. The Rangers were tenacious and highly competent soldiers and I enjoyed working with them. Unlike the Para Reg, they were a little more welcoming; however as stated earlier, no matter which unit we all were part of we were all part of a close-knit brotherhood out there and we had the right mix of blokes to do the job.

The Airborne Engineers were amazing! I saw one day they were out fortifying our positions whilst at the same time smashing the Taleban who had started firing on them! The selfless commitment to look after each other was something I hold close to my heart, every man stood up to be counted.

Bryan - this day was the day of all days in my time in Sangin, and the worst I can remember. It was the 20th August 2006. I did not get to know all the guys but had spoken to Bryan a fair few times. We had the craic about AFC Harrogate where he had previously been as an instructor but also, I was out on the ground with his section a few times and got to know them pretty well. They were a band of brothers for sure and were as tight knit as anything and with Bryan as their section commander you could tell why.

On this day there was a tasking for a platoon to provide cover for another whilst they set Bar Mines to create a route through some compounds. As normal it went tits up as the Taleban had other plans. A contact ensued and Bryan's section was forward and right at the time and they identified three enemy positions as I recall, and his section was subsequently ambushed. A lad called Briggsy was hit in the chest, but thankfully his body armour stopped the round and he continued to fight. Andy Lanaghan was hit in the face and our mate Posh Para Robbo, who was on the ground this time, was hit in the arm. The fight continued and from the rooftop we were assisting with small arms fire and artillery support whilst the platoon pulled back to the compound. It was chaos, there were the cries of "man down" on the radio but we did not know who had been hit at the time. There was utter confusion everywhere and the incoming fire from the Taleban was still ongoing. The lads were all recovered from the ground and there was a brief pause to treat our wounded and regroup. I looked down from my position and I could see that there was something not quite right. From my vantage point, I then saw a group of lads coming forward looking like they were heading back out again. I thought that this was crazy, the Company Sergeant Major (CSM) was sat on his quad bike.

I said to Jase, "something isn't right".

It was clear that someone was missing, that someone turned out to be Bryan. The lads went back out again to find him, the Taleban fire was still intense and the proximity to our guys precluded the use of artillery or close air support. Instead, Apache Helicopters were requested. More lads were injured during the rescue attempt and I remember seeing the CSM on his quad bike driving at speed in and around the compounds, yet again under fire himself searching for Bryan. He found him, he was recovered right next to three dead Taleban fighters, who he had charged down and killed to allow his own section to pull back. We did not know at the time if he was dead or alive. The last I saw of him was when the CSM drove into the compound on his quad with Bryan on top of it, he didn't look alive but there were still shouts of medic!

Bryan was pronounced dead by the Medical Officer in the Regimental Aid Post, once again, the sickness in all of our stomachs was immense. Seeing your brothers-in-arms lie there motionless is one of the most harrowing things I have ever seen and no tablets can take that away.

Bryan had done something so brave and selfless he would later be awarded the Victoria Cross (Posthumously) for his actions that day. Part of his citation reads on 20 August 2006:

'Corporal Budd was leading his section on the right forward flank of a platoon clearance patrol near Sangin District Centre. Another section was advancing with a Land Rover fitted with a .50 calibre heavy machine gun on the patrol's left flank. Pushing through thick vegetation, Corporal Budd identified a number of enemy fighters 30 metres ahead. Undetected, and in an attempt to surprise and destroy the enemy, Corporal Budd, initiated a flanking manoeuvre. However, the enemy spotted the Land Rover on the left flank and the element of surprise was lost for the whole platoon.

In order to regain the initiative, Corporal Budd decided to assault the enemy and ordered his men to follow him. As they moved forward the section came under a withering fire that incapacitated three of his men. The continued enemy fire and these losses forced the section to take cover. But Corporal Budd continued to assault on his own, knowing full well the likely consequences of doing so without the close support of his remaining men. He was wounded but continued to move forward, attacking and killing the enemy as he rushed their position.

Inspired by Corporal Budd's example, the rest of the platoon re-organised and pushed forward their attack, eliminating more of the enemy and eventually forcing their withdrawal. Corporal Budd subsequently [sic] died of his wounds, and when his body was later recovered it was found surrounded by three dead Taliban.

Corporal Budd's conspicuous gallantry during these two engagements saved the lives of many of his colleagues. He acted in the full knowledge that the rest of his men had either been struck down or had been forced to go to ground. His determination to press home a single-handed assault against a superior enemy force despite his wounds stands out as a premeditated act of inspirational leadership and supreme valour. In recognition of this, Corporal Budd is awarded the Victoria Cross."

CHAPTER 28

<u>Injuries and God</u>

I f you think I am going to preach to you from the Bible, you are mistaken but I wanted to share with you something that I have never shared with anyone apart from my wife. Without doubt my time in Sangin left its mark, physically and mentally. The constant fighting, incoming attacks, all the killed and injured will never ever leave me. My hearing was damaged in an RPG attack close to the building I was sat on and with so many close calls, I was fearing for my life, day in day out and thought there was no way I would get out alive. This was all internal thinking as externally I had to be professional, brave and help my brothers out, which I can say with conviction I did. However, at times it was that bad I resorted to prayer. My belief before being in this situation was non-committal if you like. My mum and dad had me christened as a baby and therefore I was a Christian. I never went to church on a Sunday and did not really consider having any faith up until that point. At times during a firefight or when I had a quiet moment away from the lads I would pray, and it would be a simple one. "Please God keep me alive so I can go home and see my parents, and if I am to die in this place please make it quick, Amen". As you can tell I was not used to this, but I found some relief and comfort by doing so. I do believe there is life after death and forward to 2021 I always have a robin visit my home and sit on a ceramic poppy in the garden and just wonder if the saying is true - when Robins are near, loved ones are here! And if that is any of the lads popping by to say hello.

During the battle that took Bryan's life, one of our team was hit. Posh Para Robbo had a Taleban 7.62 round straight through is arm and it was a right mess. You could see right through it! He was in so much pain and his skin had become very ashen, but he was still smoking a fag. His tour was done, and he was casevac back to Bastion, but before he did, he said to me.

"Kill the bastards for me Benny" in his very posh southern accent, as a team we did our best to oblige.

During our time in Sangin, which was just one place of many that was taking the brunt of the attacks; but as mentioned earlier in Kajaki we would hear on the radio of another incident taking place which was not through enemy action this time but just as deadly.

Mark Wright was now at Kajaki following on from his horrendous time in Sangin. It was meant to be a wind down just the same as I had experienced previously. He was there with a mortar team, snipers, and medics. On 6th September the leader of a sniper patrol, tasked with engaging a group of Taliban fighters operating on the main highway, was heading down the steep slope when he initiated a mine and sustained severe injuries.

Seeing the mine-strike from the top of the ride, Corporal Wright gathered a number of men and rushed down the slope to assist. Realising that the casualty was likely to die before a full mine clearance could be effected, Corporal Wright unhesitatingly led his men into the minefield.

Exercising effective and decisive command, he directed medical orderlies to the injured soldier, ordered all unnecessary personnel to safety, and then began organizing the casualty evacuation. He called for a helicopter and ordered a route to be cleared through the minefield to a landing site. Unfortunately the leader of this task, while moving back across the route he believed he had cleared, stepped on another mine and suffered a traumatic amputation.

Corporal Wright, again at enormous personal risk, immediately moved to the new casualty and began rendering life-saving assistance until one of the medical orderlies could take over. Calmly, Corporal Wright ordered all non-essential personnel to stay out of the minefield and continued to move around and control the incident. He sent accurate situation reports to his headquarters and ensured that additional medical items were obtained. Shortly afterwards a helicopter landed nearby but as Corporal Wright stood up, he initiated a third mine which seriously injured him and one of the orderlies. The remaining medical orderly began treating Corporal Wright but was himself wounded by another mine which caused further injury to both Corporal Wright and others. There were now seven casualties still in the minefield, three of whom had lost limbs. Despite this horrific situation and the serious injuries, he had himself sustained, Corporal Wright continued to command and control the incident. He remained conscious for much of the time, continually shouting encouragement to those around him, maintaining morale and calm amongst the many wounded men. Sadly, Corporal Wright died of his wounds on the rescue helicopter.

His supreme courage and outstanding leadership were an inspiration to his men. For acts of the greatest gallantry and complete disregard for his own safety in striving to save others, Corporal Wright is awarded the George Cross. (PARA DATA). Along with Mark's courage during the incident, I want to personally recognise all the other lads from that day who sustained life changing injuries but also the bravery of the Medic - Paul "Tug" Hartley who selflessly put himself in harm's way to treat all the injured personnel on that fateful day. Now a personal friend of mine, he is very modest in his actions, but I have no doubt at all, without his intervention and bravery, it would have been a lot worse than it already was.

Tug, as I did, enlisted in the Army straight from school following a family tradition. He joined the Royal Engineers in 1997 where he served as a systems operator until 2003 when he transferred to the Royal Army Medical Corp (RAMC) as a Combat Medical Technician, (CMT) in Afghanistan twice, Oman, Lebanon, and Canada.

Tug was awarded the George Medal (GM) for his actions during the Kajaki incident, where despite being injured himself and keeping calm in the most stressful situations, attempted to rescue and treat all the lads in the minefield and refused to stop until all were rescued and off the battlefield. Tug is an absolute gent and a hell of a rugby player that always gives of his best.

CHAPTER 29

<u>BIG PARKY 7</u>

I wanted to dedicate this chapter to one inspirational and tough individual who, despite being catastrophically injured in Afghanistan 2006, defied all the odds set against him and smashes every challenge that gets in his way. I also want to acknowledge his family Diane and Andy and the Pilgrim Bandits Charity who have been pivotal to his recovery so far and supported him with steadfast dedication throughout. The most severely injured, surviving soldier since WW2, I pay tribute to my friend Ben Parkinson MBE.

A fellow member of the Regiment is where we met. Ben is a larger than life Yorkshire man from Donny! (Doncaster) and a man mountain. He would cast a shadow when he entered the room but then would light it up with his fantastic character and personality. He was one of the good ones. We all knew how special he was, or stupid, when he attempted to pass the infamous P Company not once, nor twice but seven times, where finally he managed to become a Paratrooper. This just shows you the calibre of the man and the robustness not only of his body but his mind too. There is no bloody way I would have shown that commitment though all that torture, and that is what it was. We built up a friendship over the years and Parky would support my battery, I battery on operations in Afghanistan 2006.

Parky was a Gun Bunny or trail ape as we on the FST used to call them and was part of a Gun Crew who I mentioned earlier were integral in disrupting the Taleban and without them, the infantry units would of sustained more fatalities than they did.

(Me and Parky cutting through the ice in Greenland)

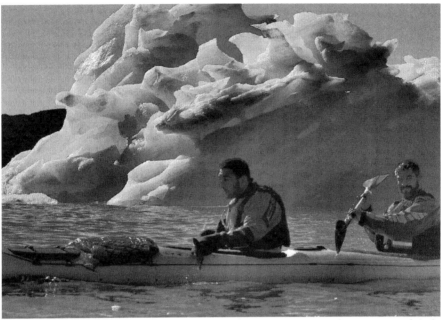

It was late on in the tour and Parky was part of a MOG, which was a mobile patrol around Helmand with the Gun Battery that could, within minutes, set up and fire on targets from their location.

I was now back at Bastion following my tour in Sangin and, selfishly I was so relieved that I was there and lived to tell the tale.

We got word that someone from the MOG had been injured, a few of us were in Bastion at the time, my buddy Babs was one of them thankfully. We hungered for news as we were aware that the MOG consisted of our Unit only.

We could not believe it, we were told it was Parky and two others, Ry Hewson, and Phil Greenaway. Parky was in the cupola of a WMICK, soft skinned land rover manning a 50-calibre machine gun.

They had accidentally driven over a soviet, anti-tank mine. Phil and Ryan were thrown clear and sustained injuries however Parky was very seriously injured and sustained multiple poly-trauma in the incident. I cannot mention certain people, as they still serve however, their actions on the ground undoubtedly saved Parky's life. They selflessly ran through the minefield to reach Ben and start treating him immediately, it was another phenomenal act of heroism of the highest order, and just shows what it means to be in this airborne brotherhood.

Babs and I went to the Med Centre at Bastion and waited for Ben to come in. He arrived back at Bastion on board the MERT (Medical Emergency Response Team) Chinook helicopter and following their interventions went straight into surgery.

We did not know at the time how bad he was and there was no one available to tell us what was going on, it was an apprehensive time.

Babs and I went back a little later to see how he was and we were told he was not in a good condition and they have had to amputate his legs. The doctors would not allow us to see him and of course, we were heartbroken, we wanted to be by his side, and we were not allowed.

Parky was flown back to Britain, I believe to allow him to die. As horrendous as that sounds, that is the feeling we had. How could he survive something like this?

He eventually landed at Birmingham Airport and I didn't know at the time, but my mum arranged the ambulance that was meeting Ben at the airport to then take him onward to Selly Oak. My Mum knew Ben and following this she could no longer bring herself to do this role.

Parky was now back in Britain and had to face many more battles from now on.

My tour in Afghanistan was over and I would never be able to shake off the horrors of it. Physically, I would never be the same nor mentally. It was the hardest thing I had ever had to face, but was nothing in comparison to those who were killed or injured, I was one of the lucky ones but had Survivor's Guilt and many other issues going on at the time but did not acknowledge them until later on.

As soon as I could I went to Selly Oak to see Ben and meet his mum, Diane. Diane is an amazing, brave, and stoic lady and a mum to us all. She fought tirelessly for Ben and others to get these injured service personnel the care they deserved and ensured that other injured servicemen and women would not have to go through the bureaucracy and bullshit Ben had to when he got back to Britain. Any way with my blood boiling, I digress.

Ben sustained horrific injuries that would have killed me and you out right, but not Ben. He broke his back, pelvis, every rib in his chest, both legs were amputated, and he had an on scene surgical airway fitted and was ventilated and the list goes on.

I walked into his room at Selly Oak Hospital and was horrified. He was in a little side room on ITU unconscious with a trachy in place, ventilating his lungs. He was in a mixed ward with folk from all walks of life which did not seem right? No military wing for our servicemen? Nope just normal service for him. I am not for one minute knocking our NHS as they did and continue to do a fantastic job, but it just seemed a little odd that Britain's most injured surviving soldier was in a bed next to Mrs Miggins and nothing was in place to support our injured servicemen and women.

I am glad to say that, in time, this all changed and in my eyes we were not expecting to see such injured people returning in this condition, this was credit to the medical staff out in Afghanistan and bringing the operating table to us in the field.

I spoke to Ben as he lay there in a coma, tried to have a laugh with him, I cried and said goodbye at the end of my first visit as I genuinely believed he would die.

He did not die! Visit after visit he showed some signs of improvement. Year after year he got stronger and stronger, and I would visit as much as I could. He did not have legs and his speech wasn't there, but I tell you what, he was still as sharp as a razor, his personality was intact and his drive to recover was there. He was picked up by Pilgrim Bandits Charity, who were set up by a group of special forces soldiers who look after military amputees. This changed Ben's life and their motto, "Always a little further" says it all. They do not do sympathy and they allow injured servicemen and women to still go out and do the things they used to do and push their limits. This charity inspired me to become a volunteer and organise events to raise awareness and funds to support not only Ben, but others who had been injured, this included Tyler, who I was in training with at Harrogate, who lost his legs in Afghanistan also. I had the opportunity to go to Greenland with Ben and be his Kayak buddy for 10 days. It was hard work but an absolute honour and a privilege to get this opportunity to support my mate in such amazing surroundings.

Ben continues to go from strength to strength but also does so much in the community supporting and inspiring others and for his charitable work, in 2015 he was awarded the MBE. I was so pleased for him and Pilgrim Bandits Charity who continue to support our injured.

Unbelievably as I have just finished writing this chapter, at 13:54 hours Tuesday 12th January 2021, Ben's mum, Diane sent me and a couple of the lads a video of him walking unaided! No sticks, no support, just him on his stubby prosthetics. This is something none of us expected to see. He has once again defied all the odds. This remarkable man was sent home to die and now I have borne witness to this! What an absolute legend, fighter and hero, I am proud to be his friend, I am proud to see his journey, and I am proud of his family. God bless you Ben Parkinson, MBE!.

"Sometimes you look at your son and just cannot believe the life that he has lived or the friends he has made". Diane said.

CHAPTER 30

From Para to Medic

We now move away from fighting on one front line to concentrate on another. The very tough transition would begin, to transform me from a soldier and everything the past seven years had taught me and the challenges I had endured, to an NHS worker on a quite different front line, back at home.

I made the decision to leave the Army whilst flying back to the UK, from Afghanistan. We stopped over in Cyprus for a few nights (decompression) which was really needed. Decompression was exactly that, a wind down and chance to catch our breath before we were to return to normality back home. We had chance to reflect on the past six months, good the bad and very ugly, we had beers (which was probably not the best idea but welcome all the same) and then got the chance to have a day on the beach, playing volleyball, messing about in the sea and just generally relaxing. This was all good, but we just wanted to get home and see our families. I spoke with the lads about how they felt and I would say 70% of them were in my camp and they would choose to leave following this tour and there was the other 30% made up of blokes who were nearly at the end of their careers or just others who clearly enjoyed it far too much and could not give up the lifestyle.

For me, up until that point, the Army was my life, and it was all I had known from 16 years old. I had done what I wanted to do, become a Paratrooper, and fought the enemy. We got to do this and some over the last six months and I will be honest, I do not believe there has been another tour as bad to date when it came to number of engagements with the enemy. Did it frighten me, the thought of going back again, potentially two or three more tours? Absolutely it did. I spent days on end being internally afraid of death or what was to come in the dynamic area I was in. Saying my prayers helped and put me at ease but I did not want to go through it again. I had given everything during my time in the military and achieved everything I wanted but at twenty-four years old, I still had lots more to experience of the world and I knew what I wanted to do, become a paramedic.

A year flew by for me preparing to leave the Army, and that is how long it takes from when you sign off on the dotted line until you are a free man. I used my time wisely taking advantage of the Army's resettlement courses to develop my knowledge.

Luckily for me I saw a job advertised with West Midlands Ambulance Service, it was not where I wanted to end up, but it was a way in and potentially a foot on the ladder in becoming a paramedic. The role was advertised as an Emergency Care Assistant or (ECA). I had never heard of such a role, I just assumed as any normal person does that anyone on an ambulance is a paramedic, but no. This was a role that was front line based but the very bottom of the pile. Without being arrogant or thinking I was some kind of war hero as I know some do, I applied and got an interview for the post.

Now going back to the Army Foundation College, Harrogate, I arrived with no grades whatsoever to my name from school, however by joining the Army and being put through different courses and gaining the skills and qualifications I did, this enabled me to get an interview, so as I said I would be forever grateful to the AFC and the Army for setting me up for a future career.

I turned up for the interview at Falcon House, Dudley (or

as some would say Dudlaaaaaaaaay) with an hour to spare, as smart as a carrot with all my documents in hand. It was clear to see from all the candidates that were there, that I was the only ex-serviceman. We stick out like a sore thumb. The military gives you confidence, good communication skills and an air around you that makes you different to the rest. The waiting room was deadly quiet, and folk were not making eye contact and I was doing my best to engage with people, and to be fair eventually started a conversation with one lad just before I got called through.

The interview was informal compared to that of the military, there was an old ambulanceman, a woman operations manager and someone from HR, all very nice and polite, once again, I was not used to this.

I answered all their questions confidently and most were around decision making and teamwork. They were probably bored of me and I reckon I sounded like Uncle Albert, "During the War" but they seemed happy. I left the interview happy and had done all I could.

I was at the time, back living with my mum and dad, which I did not mind at all, they are such fantastic people to be around. Don't get me wrong, we clashed at times as all families do, but they are always supportive, and I think they were just glad that I was home. As per my mum's statement, it was clear that I had really made them unwell, mentally, and physically due to their son being away and in danger. I played my rugby back at Willenhall at the weekends and generally mooched about waiting to see if I had got the job. I had a relationship on the go but the less said about that the better, as so many ex-serviceman and women, quite often the first serious relationship is not often the best one.

Moving swiftly on I had the phone call that I had been waiting for, I was offered the position of ECA with West Midlands Ambulance service, I was delighted.

CHAPTER 31

#AMBOLIFE

T his job is not for everyone, and in my opinion, it takes a very special somebody to become a Health Care Professional, someone that cares for each and every patient they come in to contact with; and someone that treats every patient as if it were their own flesh and blood. That is the idea anyway, however it is not always that simple when you face, violence, aggression, verbal abuse, assault, and that can just be in one shift.

I started my training to become an ECA, it was a big culture shock but I was with some great people, but as you know from courses you have been on, there is always that one knob who has either been there and done it better or knows someone who has.

In the military we had a mutual respect for each other, bonded under adversity and completed the same training. This was a completely different kettle of fish. There were people from all walks of life there. We had one lad who I won't name who was a real tool. I really did wonder how he even got the job, but these were the little things that I would really have to park if I wanted to get on well in my new job.

We had a couple of great experienced instructors who were old school and had been there and done it. They explained an overview of the training and gave us some insight how it would be out there at the coal face, working alongside Paramedics and Technicians.

In a nutshell they said that the ECA roll was not widely accepted and that the feeling among other clinicians were that we were Emergency Medical Technicians (EMT's) on the cheap. As ECAs, we had no clinical responsibility for patients and if we were to fuck up it would be on the registered paramedics shoulders.

I did feel lower than snake shit at the prospect of being the new lad again, I had been through it before, knew how it felt and just could not be bothered with it, I had to try though. I needed to recognise that the past was just that and nobody owed me anything, not even respect for fighting for the country. There was a part of me that just wanted mutual, professional respect, if that was the case, I would be happy.

We had a good time during our training, and we covered theoretical and practical assessment in, Basic Life Support, (BLS), manual handling, assisting the Paramedic as well as extremely basic techniques like airway management, controlling bleeding and medical emergencies.

I really got into it and enjoyed learning more about the human body, treatment, and the theory behind it. As I said this was all extremely basic but as in the military, I wanted to be the best I could with whoever I worked with and to do my best for the patients I would meet.

The training flew by and we passed all our assessments. On the last day, the instructors told us to assemble downstairs outside the building we were training in. I thought 'what's going on here?'. Outside were parked two minibuses. we were told to get on there, and we did just that! On we jumped and set off down the road into Brierly Hill High Street, it was packed as normal, market stalls open and the streets were crammed with shoppers. We were not told anything until we pulled up in a bus stop, brakes slammed on and one of the instructors jumped out and made his way around to the back doors. They flung the back doors open:

"Right, you lot, male collapsed in the street, go and sort it out". He said.

What the hell was he on about? Had he brought us out on an actual working job? As I jumped out, I could see a manikin on the footpath with a bag of medical equipment at the side of it and members of the public just looking at us like we were mad.

There was obvious hesitation, but the instructor said again.

"Well come on then he doesn't look very well, get on with it".

With that, we all piled out of the bus and thankfully, I was with some of the good guys, and we all worked as a team to sort out the problem. We had to get stuck into this roleplay. Are we in any danger? responses? the standard question "hello sir, can you hear me?" Airway, breathing and circulation, each one of these we had to assess quickly and decide on the best course of action. In this case it was a Cardiac Arrest, quickly identifiable we cracked on and commenced Basic Life Support, (BLS) which for us was no different than a normal bystander. Identify as above that they were unresponsive and not breathing normally, or not breathing at all, call for help and commence Cardio Pulmonary Resuscitation, (CPR) which in basic terms is chest compressions at a rate of thirty compressions to two rescue breaths. For us at the time we had our own pocket mask that we would place over the patient's mouth and nose and blow into it, but thankfully the evidence now shows compression only CPR is adequate. We were to continue this until senior help arrived. We were able to use Automated External Defibrillators (AED) which were simple bits of kit, two pads one on the top left of the patient's chest and one on the right flank then just follow the instructions. We had all this going on, on the High Street with an audience so it was to put a little pressure on us, and I really did enjoy it. It was not real, and was all set up; however, some elements were really good, and always a key point was to expect the unexpected.

It did worry me a little though when an old girl passed us and said "He dow look very well he dow?" in a broad, black country accent, it did make me smile. Training done, I am now an ECA and for the next stage I would have to complete my Emergency Blue Light course.

Four weeks of razzing round in an ambulance sounds good, right? If only! This course was harder than the medical part of our training. My instructor was Calvin Ward, who was a top bloke and another old school ambulance man who had been there and done it. He was missing a digit on his hand. "How you lose that Calvin?" I asked him.

"Bloody student took the corner too fast, tipped the ambulance and I got my fingers trapped in the door, so don't get any ideas". He returned.

Over the next four weeks we would have to learn the Highway Code off-by-heart and make note of all of our exemptions we could use when driving on blue lights. It was bloody exhausting, the days were long, although we did get to drive out to places like the Great Orme, near Llangollen, Wales which is a beautiful place.

Our motto or key phrase throughout the whole of the course was IPGSA. This bloody mnemonic used to get on my tits! To this day I still can reel it off any time I want. It stood for, Information, position, gear, speed, acceleration. This, in a nutshell, was emergency driving, we had to give regular commentary on what we could see, looking near, middle, and far, while negotiating hazards. It was so tiring.

Eventually following an intense three weeks we were allowed to drive under emergency conditions. A skill that would be an integral part of my role on an ambulance. It is not about getting to the emergency as fast as you can, as some people think, it's about driving to arrive safely and efficiently. Now as I had operated in some hostile areas in the past with stresses that others may not have faced, I took to the driving calmly and proficiently. Some of the morons had a problem with always seeing red mist, their vision and judgement were impaired, and you could say they were a bit excitable. They would throw the ambulance left right and Chelsea, without any consideration for the people in the rear, they soon got told!

CHAPTER 32

<u>Roles</u>

As above I mentioned I started as an ECA, this role was the very lowest rung on the ladder. Previously on a front-line ambulance there had ever only been paramedics and EMTs, so my new role was not very well received. My very first posting was to Bristol Road Ambulance Station, Birmingham. I was really apprehensive about my first day, it was new, and I had to start from the bottom. In my head I had a plan to go in, introduce myself, keep my mouth shut and be as helpful as I could be to whoever I worked with. I arrived early on my first day, parked the car up and approached the front of the station. As I got to the door, I looked through the window and the mess room was full, I thought shit, all eyes will be on me. I had no codes or any clue what I was doing which added to the anxiety. I rang the bell and a tall chap with glasses approached. He opened the door.

"Hello, I'm Dave, new ECA here for my first day".

This Twat who I can't name returned with.

"Oh, another fucking ECA to carry our kit".

My blood boiled and that was the first person I had met from station, somehow, I held my tongue and thankfully was then met by Amita the Station Manager who was lovely.

We had a chat and she showed me around and introduced me

to some of the guys and girls who were there and in fairness, they were friendly and welcoming. This chap who was off with me I would soon learn was a bad egg and had nothing to fear from him.

I cracked on around station, looking around, familiarising myself with it all and just kept myself to myself. I interacted when I needed too and was the grey man, like in the military. I asked if people wanted a brew and just made myself useful. It was important to me that I settled in and got a good reputation and as my first couple of station induction days came to an end, I felt a little easier in myself. This twat kept having digs at me and was clearly trying to test me out in front of others. He called me things like clinical waste and driver. It got my back up and he was the only one who seemed to have a problem with me. I did a week on station initially from Monday to Friday, learning about policy, procedures etc, and was told that the following week, I would get to go out on an ambulance as third man on a crew. This is what I wanted and was really excited about it. It was around finish time for me at the end of a busy induction week, and I got my things and left the building, without realising the chap who had given me shit all week followed behind. His car was parked near mine.

This time he saw me and funnily enough, did not give me any stick as there was only me and him there. I put my things in the car and approached him. He looked very sheepish as I approached, I wanted to clear the air with this individual as I could not be doing with this every shift.

"What's your problem"? I asked.

Now I don't know if it was my demeanour or body language, but he shit himself.

"I haven't got a problem". He replied in his now squeaky voice.

"You have given me nothing but shit for a week and I want to know why, you're a fucking bully!" I told him.

"I'm just trying to be funny" he returned.

He could see it in my eyes that I did not find it funny at all, and I felt I needed to nip this in the bud quickly. If I had not, it could have got out of hand.

"You aren't funny, no one else was laughing and it is becoming personal, if it happens again next week, you can fucking stand by, son" I returned.

Yes, I called him son, I could have knocked him spark out where he stood the smug little prick! How dare he treat new staff like he had? But I tell you what, he didn't do it again! This would be the first of many interactions with people who I felt treated me poorly, just because of the role I was doing. I would never have treated people like this and that was the difference.

My mum and dad brought me up to treat as you want to be treated and through my military career and while still upholding their values, I always tried to bring them into the civilian world and nine times out of ten, they worked.

I was now a civilian ambulanceman and I had to realise that people by my side are not those like in Afghanistan, who had my back no matter what, out here there were snakes in the grass, and I had to tread carefully.

Over the next few weeks, I completed numerous observations shifts and got into a routine of how the job worked. I was soon out on the road working alongside a paramedic and did my best to support them as best as possible. There were many firsts for me during the first few months of my new job. A first Cardiac Arrest, a first Myocardial Infarction (MI) and everything else in between. I was a go-for, fetch this, do that, bring me this, drive here, it was a steep but very enjoyable start, but I always knew I wanted to do more. Yes, I had been on these types of jobs and got to do CPR on the elderly and drive to hospital quickly with critically ill patients on board, but it was not enough.

I built up a good reputation and staff were fond of me and knew I was good to work with. I did as I was told, tried to pre-empt things and be an efficient member of the team. The staff on my station built up their trust in me and I had no issues there at all after that.

Sometimes though I was required to work from other stations in Birmingham and something magical and mysterious used to happen. The station manager would call someone who I was meant to be working with on a different station, as they were single manned, and by the time I had drove over to crew up with them, they would have vanished, just like magic, the reason for this was that they clearly did not want to work with an ECA as that would mean they would actually have to do their job for the day and wouldn't get to drive!!.

This was not said for all, but it just highlighted how selfish and lazy some staff were. I found it frustrating and pathetic. I wanted to move closer to home, back to Wolverhampton so put a transfer request in as soon as I could. Nearly a year went by and I was getting more and more experience and had to deal with some pretty bad things including hangings, murders, road traffic collisions and I handled it extremely well. I managed to separate myself from the jobs as I was not really hands-on at times, and up to that point had seen far worse at war. I got my transfer and went home, my new base was Penn Ambulance station, Wolverhampton.

CHAPTER 33

Ambo Family

I had landed back at home. Penn station was a very friendly place with some amazing people based there. I felt thankful for the move back and I could now help people in my local community. Penn Station was tiny, three ambulance bays, a small office and a cosy messroom. The messroom on an ambulance station is the most important room of all. It is a place where over the years you will, eat, laugh, cry, celebrate New Year and everything else. It will be your counselling room and your colleagues are the medication. It is the focal point for all staff where anything goes, a sacred place. This is the first time I got to have some continuity, I got a shift place and worked with some real characters. Neil Weaver, (Weave), Dave Facey, (Face-ache) and Alistair McNeil, all paramedics, and all very different personalities. On one 12-hour shift on an ambulance there is that much that happens, but I want to tell you about a few things that we faced together during my time at Penn.

Weave and I signed on for the night shift and dead on 18:00 we got our first job. We would not likely now see base again until tomorrow morning so we would make the most of it. With the vehicle partly checked we went off to a run of the mill job. An old boy with cardiac chest pain. We got a good history, completed all his checks, blood pressure, twelve lead ECG, blood sugar, oxygen saturations, had a listen to his chest and treated him at the time with Aspirin and GTN (Glyceryl Trinitrate) which is a vasodilator which widens the blood vessels. Now before that can be given, we need to ask if a patient has taken Sildenafil (Viagra) as to not drop his blood pressure. This old boy was sat in his pants on the edge of his bed, unkempt and obviously not looking after himself, which is all part of our assessment, to ensure he has the right care in place.

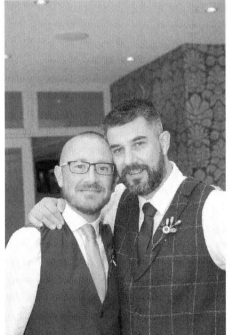

(Me and Weave, later he would become my Best Man)

"Yow had any Viagra bud before I give u a spray of this" we asked him. This is how we asked as we had already built up that rapport with him, we had a laugh and a chat and that put him at ease. As ambulance staff, that is a gift and if you can talk to patients from all walks of life, you have cracked it.

"What do yow think? I'm shagging all the time, I cor bloody breathe for one" he joked.

We all laughed together, this was typical type of banter between crew and patient and I loved this side of the job. Weave took me under his wing. He was older than me but turned out we attended the same High School and we had lots in common. We would socialise on our days off and become the best of mates. I trusted him completely as he did me. He mentored me and finally I got an opportunity to do my EMT ticket which I was really chuffed with. It would give me the chance to make decisions on patients and treat them on my own, which is what I wanted to do all along.

During another night shift with Weave, we were shattered. We had been run ragged all night and it must have been around 04:00am and we were tasked to an overdose at Heath Town Flats, Wolverhampton, a deprived area of the city.

We arrived at the address not knowing how we had got there we were that tired, and we got out of the truck to go and find this male who had apparently taken an overdose. We could hear some crashing and banging just in front of us and Weave and I looked at each other and knew that this was our patient. He lived on the 3rd floor and was currently emptying the contents of his flat, over the balcony on to the ground in front of us. There were TVs, mattresses, a fish tank, and everything else you could imagine.

"I cannot be arsed with this, can you?" I said to Weave.

Not at all, we knew it would be a ball ache. Of course, there were no police around to help us which was not unusual, and we made our way up three flights of stairs to see how we could assist this chap.

We gingerly poked our heads round his door.

"Hello Ambulance" we called.

"Fuck off "he replied, once again, not unusual.

We shined a torch in to have a look at him. He was about forty years old, just had his underwear on and that was it. What we did spot, though, was a kitchen knife in his hand.

"For fuck's sake mate, we going to have to call the police" Weave said to me, so I did I put a call in.

What were we going to do? We needed to get him to put the knife down before we do anything. We had to decide if we were going to walk away due to the danger to us, at the same time thinking what is best for him. Clearly, he needed some help. We looked from where we were, and we did not have any quick escape routes. If he went for us, we would have to drop kit and run. At this stage, the patient could see us talking.

"Fuckin help me I want to die"!

"Mate we can't help you if you got that knife in your hand, can we?" we replied.

"Come and take it off me". He replied.

There was no chance of this happening and we were not sure what he was going to do. This may sound quite scary to some, but ambulance crews faced this daily, and it was not a new thing. Weave and I were very street wise and knew the craic, some younger more inexperienced clinicians may have done things differently. The patient was trying to scare us.

"Look mate, we want to help you, but you have to help yourself, put the knife down and come and talk to us!" I reasoned with him.

He did and it seemed far too easy. Then, he came towards us and we still managed to maintain a non-threatening posture so as not to intimidate him. We locked his door popped a blanket on him and he seemed compliant. As we started walking down towards the ambulance, he went from 0 -100 in aggression towards us, throwing a melee of punches towards us. We could not run, and we had to try our best to restrain him using the techniques we had been taught but we were blowing. He had some real strength but eventually we managed to grip him. It was scary and unpredictable and luckily Weave and I knew what to expect. This was a job at 04:00am in the morning when me, Weave or the patient could have been seriously injured. You must be ready for anything when working on the front line and is just one example of the violence we faced daily.

CHAPTER 34

Stand Clear!

Plodding along and learning from the good people I worked with and ignoring some of the bad thing's others were doing seemed to be the theme. The likes of Weave and Alister were great role models for me, hugely different in many ways with different ways of working but no matter, the patient was always at the centre of the care and that is all that matters.

One evening I was working with Alister from Penn station but this time I was a fully qualified EMT. Following passing my course there was a probation period where we had to be signed off in different areas such as Basic Life Support, Childbirth etc. Obviously, you cannot predict what jobs will come up so some of them had to be done as an exercise or OCSCE.

We got a call from a patient with chest pains and made our way to the job. There seemed to be nothing out the ordinary as chest pain is a very common occurrence but this one was going to be very different.

We arrived at the address where we found a forty-year-old bloke sat in his chair in his living room. From first impressions, he looked ok, he was not sweaty, a little ashen and just a little uncomfortable. Once again, we do all his observations which included twelve lead ECG which are really detailed and look at the heart from all different angles, allowing diagnosis of certain conditions. Paramedics are trained to work through the twelve lead ECGs systematically. The ECG looks at the electrical activity in three orthogonal directions, right-left, superior-inferior, anterior and posterior, believe me it may sound complicated and for me it was, some pick it up straight away but for me I really had to work for it.

We got a history from the patient and from that and his ECG it appeared that it was in a grey area, some cardiac symptoms and some muscular skeletal. We treated for the worse of the two and recommended he come into hospital with us for a check-up.

Like I said a fairly run of the mill job. We got a chair for him, so as not to put any more strain on his heart, if that was the cause and got him settled onto the stretcher on the back of the ambulance. what happened next was a first for me.

The patient's daughter was at the rear of the ambulance.

"Will you go and fetch me my slippers bab?" he asked her.

Off she went and I shut the rear of the doors and Alister jumped in the front ready to set off.

I placed all our monitoring equipment back on this gent and started to do some paperwork. All the sudden, his movements caught my eye, both his arms went straight down his body, his head and neck arched back, and he went ridged. The colour drained from his face, which happened all within a matter of seconds, I thought -what the hell is going on, run of the mill chest pain? I glanced over my shoulder to see what was happening on the monitor, and his normal run of the mill ECG was no more. He was in Ventricular Fibrillation (VF). Shit! He was having a Cardiac Arrest, right here, right now in front of me on my first shift as a qualified EMT. VF is an abnormal heart rhythm in which the ventricles of the heart quiver instead of pumping as normal. They teach you to check the airway and breathing. No time for that this time! I did check his pulse and he did not have any. I checked on his neck (carotid) and wrist (radial). I reached into the top pouch of the monitor, grabbed the defibrillator pads, ripped the leads off his chest I had placed earlier and slapped on the pads, one top left of his chest, the other on the right side of his chest. It all happened so quickly, and I recognised it early enough to react. I charged the defibrillator and by this time Allister was alongside me thankfully.

"Charging" I called, "stand clear".

I delivered the shock. Some people may think that they jump ten feet off the ground when they receive a shock. This is not the case. There is an instant, aggressive twitch but that is it. From this point I re-checked to see if he had a pulse, to my relief he did. Allister and I set to work again and assessed his airway and breathing and got a new ECG prepared. This patient was moaning for a few minutes and still unconscious, but alive and breathing. After around two or three minutes he started to come around.

"How you are doing mate? You Ok?" I asked.

"Yeah, I am ok, what's happened?" he said.

"You just had a bit of a funny turn mate, but you're ok now" I said.

You look back now and this man had just died right in front of us, had we not of acted in the way we did, he would have died and potentially would not have been saved. He was in the absolute best place and we used defibrillation to get his heart back into sync, it was fate, he felt unwell, called the ambulance, everything looked normal and that happened anyway.

His daughter came back with his slippers.

"Everything ok?" she asked.

"Yeah, yeah, no problems at all, we are going to get him in on blue lights, but please don't worry, it's just busy in the traffic and we don't want him to wait."

This was blatant lies, but you know what? Sometimes needs must. The patient was back in the room and we knew the best place for him. A scary moment for me but I did well. Allister was supportive and praised my actions. If only all the cardiac arrests I would attend in the future ended like this, I am afraid to say they didn't.

CHAPTER 35

<u>Paramedic Dave</u>

I enjoyed my time as an ECA and EMT, but the ownership of the incidents were not mine. I had been to some nasty jobs but always had a paramedic holding my hand to take the pressure off. I wanted to do more and be able to deliver more lifesaving skills to my patients. I was lucky I had the chance to work alongside Alister and Weave who were mentors to me, but adversely to that I was sick to death of working with idiots who looked down on me.

There were many occasions when I was spoken to like an idiot, more so than when I was a soldier. The one day, I attended a job and as luck should have it, I knew the family, and had done all my life. The Crew mate I was on with at the time, a paramedic with little man syndrome took an opportunity to belittle me in front of the family, just to get a rise. They knew me, so instantly I had a rapport with them which really got the angry little man's back up. We had to do a few observations on a patient and before I got stuck in. This bell-end I was working with said:

"This is Dave, he has no clinical responsibility, and he needs to practice observations, are you happy for him to proceed?"

What a prick! There was absolutely no need at all. He made me so angry and embarrassed in front of the family. He was a Manc who had been in the RAF, and he really boiled my piss this day. Professionally I cracked on with the job and waited for the opportunity to tune him in.

Trust is a massive thing on an ambulance, and you must have each other's back all the time, in decision making, safety and just in general. I did not trust him as far as I could throw him. We got back to the ambulance and he tried to take the keys off me to drive.

"Give me the keys then" he said,

"You can fuck right off" I replied, "you just embarrassed me in front of this family, you said I had no clinical responsibility and now you want to swan about and drive all day, I think fuckin not" I returned.

He knew his cards were marked, he was another bully, and it did not wash with me. He was the type of paramedic who thought he was better than everyone else and in fact, he was the worst of them. People like him who complete inappropriate assessments and have a bad attitude were dangerous but the one night I did have to laugh.

We turned up at a job where a lorry had hit a pedestrian with its wing mirror. It was a glancing blow, and all was well, apart from an irate bloke who wanted the lorry driver's head. This idiot I was working with went full steam into the situation as normal and approached this already furious gent, "Fella! If you don't calm down, I'll put you down". He shouted.

This was music to my ears. We were on the back of the Ambulance at the time and this bloke grabbed hold of this idiot I was working with and threw him all over the ambulance, it was a delightful sight.

"Dave, help me "He was shouting.

I was pissing myself; little bully boy was getting taught a lesson.

Finally, after it all calmed down and tears were pouring down his face he asked,

"Why didn't you help me Dave",

"You really need to ask me that?" I returned bluntly. "you're a bully and I do not trust you; you have no respect for me, and I will not support a bully!"

From this day funnily enough, no more dramas with him. It was my time to set my own path and become a paramedic.

I did well as an EMT but now was time to step up and get my ticket. We had to go for a selection for a thirty two-week EMT-Paramedic course. I did well and was offered a place. On my course with me was a beautiful woman called Rhoda, who years later would become my wife and mother of my wonderful three boys, so yes that's the happy ending. I found University hard. We studied at Birmingham City University and had lectures, essays and practical assessments as well as allocated placements back on ambulances to practice the trade, as they say. I did not enjoy the theoretical side, although important, I needed to be out there helping real people in their time of need.

I did not wish as some do for blood and guts, I simply wanted to use my skills to make a difference. Fast forward a little, we qualified with commendations from our course, Rhoda and I were now a couple and we really bounced off each other and I felt really supported and comfortable in her presence.

Now a registered Paramedic, it was all on me, from having someone holding my hand and supporting me, the buck now stopped with me and I had to support more junior staff and I would not treat them as I was treated that's for sure.

CHAPTER 36

The Reality of it all

B eing a shift worker on an ambulance is really hard work. I did twelve-hour shifts both days and nights and it does really take its toll on your body and mind. On a day shift say 06:00- 18:00 you would turn up half hour early to relieve the night crew who would look like death warmed up. They looked pale, shattered, and demoralised. If we were lucky, we would have time for a brew and to check the ambulance for all the essential kit. Before checks are completed, you are out the door on your first call, more than likely not to return to station again for the rest of the day.

Not every job you would attend in a twelve-hour shift is life threatening. You may go days without seeing anything like that, but rest assured, you will see it. I had seen friends killed, I killed the enemy in Afghanistan and before joining the ambulance service I would say I had seen it all. I had not and the horrors that were in front of me as a paramedic would never go away.

Day to day you would race through the traffic on blue lights to chest pains, breathing difficulties, falls, overdoses, everything you can think of but then out the blue you are sent jobs that are a little out the ordinary that you may have to think a little differently about.

I recall one morning, I booked on the rapid response vehicle RRV as my crewmate for the day was off sick and I just made a brew, my radio went off, strange I thought, what do they want this early?

"RP252"

"Thanks Dave sorry to start your day off like this but we have a possible male hanging in Penn, Wolverhampton, I will send it through now".

Great! I thought. I was only recently qualified there were no other crews anywhere in sight and now it was time to step up. I am not going to lie, if confirmed, this would be the first hanging I would have attended alone. I was extremely nervous on the inside but calm on the outside. I set off on the short journey down the road.

I pulled into the street, parked up and grabbed my monitor, Basic Life Support kit (BLS), Advanced Life Support (ALS) kit and everything I would potentially need for this type of job. I was met by a woman, who looked uneasy, I think she was a neighbour and she pointed me towards the address.

I could hear a male's voice shouting, 'No, nooooo' which sent a shiver down my spine. I walked through the house and out to the back garden, at that point I saw a young male hanging by his neck by some blue rope, attached to an oak tree on the other side of a fence. The screams and the atmosphere were horrendous. As I approached the fence I needed to negotiate, there was a thud, the young lad had been cut down, and now lay motionless.

I got over the fence there was a distraught gentleman.

"Who is he?" I asked him gently.

"It's my son" he replied.

He was beside himself and so distressed, helpless, and scared. I cannot imagine what was going through his mind. I knelt by the side of his son and assessed him for signs of life, but it was obvious, he was dead. He was freezing cold to touch, cyanosed (blue) and bloated in the face and rigor mortis (stiffness) and hypostasis (blood draining to limbs under gravity) was present in his lower limbs. He had probably been there for around eight hours listening to the history. The son had long brown hair and colourful tattoo sleeves on both arms. His father pleaded with me to do something, which I totally understand. There was noise coming from his airway and he presumed he was breathing, tragically, he wasn't. The father was angry and frustrated, but it was clear there was nothing that could be done. I had to be empathetic but stern.

"I am very sorry, your son is dead, there is nothing I can do." I said.

There can be no mixing words or giving false hope, that was it. My hands on his shoulders and looking at him straight in the eye was the way it had to be done this time round. With the uniform and my confident approach, he accepted what he did not want to accept, the anger and frustration became hurt and he began to weep uncontrollably. His son would have been about eighteen years of age, and it was an awful incident to be involved in. Myself, the father and this young lad were stood under the tree where he had chosen to take his life and I felt sad for the father. He would have to live with this for the rest of his life. At this stage, the ambulance turned up who were sent to support me. They asked if I needed anything and all I wanted was a blanket. They went and fetched me one and passed it over the fence. I once again knelt next to the body, shut his eyes which were fixed and dilated and draped a blanket over his head and body, the father had seen enough.

Back then, we had to do an ECG trace of all the deceased and as expected the rhythm was a flat wavy line, known as asystole. We could not lift the fence panel, so we helped the father over the fence and back into his house. He was beside himself which again changed to numbness, the first and most important thing we did for him, was put the kettle on.

That was a horrendous job and one of many that followed over the years that I was glad was now behind me. Hangings are not things to witness, they are quite medieval in nature but over the years I would see many more unfortunately along with other types of suicide and trauma. Hangings do not go away as other jobs do, and I remember them all vividly. That was another bit of mental health that we put in our rucksack that day, hoping it never gets full. With Iraq and Afghanistan and a few years in the ambulance service, the rucksack was filling up quickly and once filled we all know what happens, the contents pour out onto the floor.

CHAPTER 37

<u>A Brew and a chat</u>

This is how we deal with a nasty incident, a brew, and a chat. One thing I believe all Ambulance Trusts do well is look after their own. Following a traumatic incident, I have always found the welfare to be brilliant. That one job I mentioned, a young lad hanging did not just affect his family but also affected the lady in the Emergency Operations Centre (EOC) who answered the call, it affected me and the ambulance crew, the neighbour of the family involved, all within a short space of time and we need to recognise this.

The men and women of the EOC do an amazing job in such a pressurised environment. They have people abusing them on the call, have death threats and must take calls for the most traumatic and upsetting of incidents. On top of this that day they had to make sure I was OK.

Following this job, I was ok, all I wanted was five minutes to myself and a brew, just to pack all my equipment away and have a breather. The best type of counselling I have ever had come in the form of having a chat in the mess room. This was a sacred time where you would get to have a brew, discuss the job, what went well, what didn't, your colleagues and managers would always be one hundred percent supportive and would always manage to cheer you up and get you recharged and ready to go again. The majority of the time this would involve piss-taking so if you have no sense of humour, I am afraid this isn't the job for you.

Over the years this was the way and following a bad job an informal debrief followed by a brew was enough. The things you see and hands on involved in being a front line paramedic you would not believe, but there is no one else and we were there at the worse point in people's lives, just to pick up the pieces, literally at times, and make everything better. This is a big responsibility and one I enjoyed doing.

As a paramedic working in Wolverhampton, my colleagues and I had seen it all. It was a dynamic environment to work in and that was the exciting bit, you never knew what would come next.

So, following a nasty job, a brew, and a chat it was time to crack on with the shift. Your last job could have been death and destruction but the next one could be an absolute pile of shit. For example, and in the nicest possible way, we are all not born intelligent, for some they will never reach dizzy intellectual heights. All of you reading this would only dream of calling 999 if there was a true threat to life. Not everyone who lived in our wonderful city would do the same.

Down the road from the ambulance station was a well-known family, they would call an ambulance every single day for either a chest pain, overdose or whatever they could think of at the time. We obviously had to respond and year after year we would know them personally, they would know us, they would wave to you when we were off duty, it was a love hate relationship. In the early days you get frustrated with these 'regulars' or 'frequent flyers' as they would waste ambulance time. Eventually you end up taking no notice and getting in and out as quick as possible, making sure they were ok but freeing yourself up so that you could respond to more appropriate calls.

People say to us all the time 'I bet you see some sights' the same old shit statement that you would ask a taxi driver. 'Have you been busy? 'What time do you finish?' but the one time my crewmate and I that evening did see some sights when we visited our regular family.

It was late evening and we had the inevitable call to see the head of this family with chest pains. Off we trotted down the road, I remember it being a weekend night.

"I bet they are all pissed up" I said to Mick, as they loved a drink and not only at the weekend.

We grabbed our kit and walked into the property. It was a shit-hole complete with sticky carpets and the smell of cat piss. You wouldn't sit down and have a brew with them, and it was that type of house that you wipe your feet on the way out.

We were led upstairs to a back bedroom and were told:

"He's in there".

I can remember hearing some moaning and groaning, just presumed it was the patient, Mick and I entered the room, and the stench was horrific. There was the patient in the room, smoking of course but he was not alone. He was in the room with his son and a woman, and they were not shy or bothered in the very slightest that we were there. The moaning and groaning were coming from them! To our surprise and disgust this couple were shagging on a sofa in the corner of the room!

"Sorry to ruin the party guys, but can you take it elsewhere whilst we sort the patient out" I said to them.

Yes, I could have chosen my words a little better, granted, but we were met with:

"Fuck off we are nearly done".

Honestly, Wolverhampton's finest. You could not make things up on this job, you really do see it all and I can honestly say nothing ever surprises me.

I had a very good few years in Wolverhampton, managed to save a few lives, help bring new life into the world and every time I did, I made sure I asked the couple, "are you going to call it Dave?" Fortunately, to my knowledge none of them did. We worked with the Police and the Fire Service at Road Traffic Collisions, resuscitated people from burning buildings and I learnt a lot in a short space of time. In this job you are either a "Shit

189

Magnet" or not, some staff never have bad jobs, and some get them all the time, it is just luck of the draw.

Not content with how I was progressing I wanted more, and my next ambition was to become a HART Paramedic. I know what you are thinking, a paramedic that knows lots about hearts! Not at all! I was shortlisted for selection on to the Hazardous Area Response Team (HART) based at Oldbury in the Heart of the Black Country.

CHAPTER 38

<u>HART LIFE</u>

The HART was a new concept in terms of ambulance work, here is a little history lesson.

The 7th July 2005 is a day we will never forget as 52 people in London lost their lives, 700 more injured. On the morning commute to work for many in central London, four suicide bombers set about inflicting terror on the capital bringing everything to a halt. Attacks on the London Underground and on buses ensured that sheer panic ensued. This was a well organised, coordinated attack and at the time there were Police, Fire and Ambulance staff along with many civilians bravely running towards the danger in an attempt to save as many lives as possible. The HART concept came about shortly after these horrific attacks and would later allow paramedics to specialise in certain areas and enable them to operate and save more life within the "HOT ZONE" of a major incident.

Hazardous Area Response Teams – more commonly known as HART – are comprised of specially recruited personnel who are trained and equipped to provide the ambulance response to high-risk and complex emergency situations.

HART teams are based in each of England's ten NHS Ambulance Trusts, which means they can cover the whole of the country, in some cases working together on specific, large scale or high-profile incidents, either accidental or deliberately caused.

HART teams work alongside the police and fire & rescue services within what is known as the 'inner cordon' (or 'hot zone') of a major incident. The job of the HART teams is to triage and treat casualties and to help save in exceedingly difficult circumstances.

They are also there to look after other emergency personnel who may become injured whilst attending these difficult and challenging incidents.

HART teams are tactically capable of responding to the following types of challenging incident:

Hazardous Materials – Working inside the inner cordon where hazardous materials are present; dealing with the aftermath of industrial accidents; transporting patients with high-risk infectious diseases, for example Ebola; undertaking complex transportation cases (for example, after large scale accidents).

CBRN(e) – Chemical, Biological, Radiological, Nuclear and Explosives – Providing the NHS specialist healthcare inner cordon response to CBRN(e) events.

MTA – Marauding Terrorist Attack – Providing the NHS specialist healthcare response to acts of terrorism involving explosive devices, firearms, knives and / or weaponised vehicles.

SWAH – Safe Working at Height – Providing the specialist healthcare response to patients taken ill at height, either on man-made structures or within the natural environment.

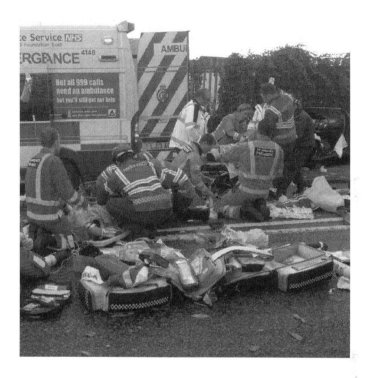

(Teamwork ,D Team assisting with a Complex, life threatening road traffic collision RTC, with multiple critically injured patients)

Confined Spaces – Providing the specialist healthcare response to patients caught in substantially enclosed spaces; following building collapses; where compromised atmospheres are present, where entrapment of patients is hampering the delivery of care.

Unstable Terrain – Providing the specialist healthcare response to patients caught within active rubble piles or where rural access or difficult terrain is providing a specific challenge to the rescue and extrication effort.

Water Operations – Providing the specialist healthcare response to patients caught in water environments, for example swift water rescue, or where urban or rural flooding has occurred, and including deployment to boat operations.

Providing support to security operations – Providing healthcare support to specific Government security operations, support to police operations such as incidents where illicit drug laboratories are present, and VIP close protection support (naru.org.uk)

This is a very specialist role and luckily, I was successful at the selection day and at interview. That was the easy bit, the tough stuff was to come. With all those types of incidents mentioned above, I would experience all of them in some way shape or form over the next three years. Looking back now the three years spent on this specialist team were the best of my ambulance career so far and I can put that down to one thing- D Team, what a fantastic bunch of lads to serve with I will talk more about that motley crew soon.

Along with all the other successful recruits we had a year of tough training in front of us, physical and mentally tough. We would complete the Fire and Rescue Service Breathing apparatus course which was three weeks and would enable us to operate using extended duration breathing apparatus (EDBA) for use in contaminated environments such as fires or chemical incidents. This was a very demanding course along with the swift water rescue course which would allow us to operate near or in swift water. The training was second to none, unlike the military we had access to all the latest equipment and the best training available, this was completely different to the normal ambulance service where you would get one mandatory update per year.

It meant lots of time away from home for the first year but the satisfaction I got on completion was immense, I was now a fully trained HART Operative.

CHAPTER 39

D Team

I was so proud to be part of this Team first and foremost, we would now work together for the next 3 years. On reflection, it was not always easy to get along, we argued, we laughed, and we cried but we always did the job well. We spent more time with each other than we did with our own family and to this day I call them all brothers as I did with the Military lads. Over the three years we would face some really tough times together. We would have to watch each other's backs, support each other mentally and physically in testing situations to come. A brief introduction to the team, our glorious Team Leader was Ed Middleton, a Staffordshire lad and ex Light Infantry Soldier, he was a highly experienced paramedic, a fitness fanatic and all-round good lad. He was a good man manager, switched on and new when to have a laugh and knew when to switch it on. We all followed by his example and stupidly followed him when he had some crazy fitness idea or "fun game "to play.

Olly Ayles was a Shropshire lad who had hollow legs and could eat like a lion and the man we looked up to for the clinical knowledge and direction. He was a really intelligent man who did need his coffee in a morning to get him rocking and rolling, a little bit grumpy first thing and could not be doing with our antics early in the morning. He was Mr dependable as always which can be said for all these guys. We had Chris Harte (Mini) or over the years (not so mini) wind up merchant who I completed my paramedic course with. He was a lovely lad apart from being born in Birmingham, who at times (do not get me wrong) I could have beaten to death when he comes out with some smart comment but all the same great, dependable lad to be around. Neil Baars, (Baarsy), was a Bromsgrove lad who was also really experienced and had been a paramedic for a long while out in the shires. He, too, was a rugby lad who could also turn his hand to anything, a really creative character who spoke lots of sense and played the saxophone on a night. Last but not least was Millie Millward who was the heart of the team. He was from Malvern and spoke like a farmer. Hilarious! Millie was a kind character who would always get the job done. You could always rely on him to come out with an awkward statement. You will find out more about these amazing guys as we go on.

Our normal run of shifts on HART were two days and two nights, based in Oldbury in the Black Country. The routine was vastly different to being on a front-line ambulance. We would not have to rush out first thing and we would not get battered for 12 hours bouncing from one job to the next, but if we did deploy to a job, it potentially could be very protracted due to the nature of it.

We had lots of equipment to check daily from our EDBA that I mentioned earlier. Our drugs to sign out, Morphine and Diazimuls and vehicle equipment checks. During the day there was always things to do on station. We were extremely fortunate that there was a gym, and we had the time to use it. Some days would pass, and we would not get tasked to a job but then others you are out all day. Night shifts, I am not going to lie, you could get some head down when all the work was done and in fairness, the situations we found ourselves in at times, you needed the prior rest. I want to share with you some of the incidents we attended together as a team to give you a flavour of what it was like in a team at some of the more disturbing incidents. Believe me, this is not to make the read sexier, just to show what we were involved in and the mechanisms that affected us following them.

Suicides were a fairly frequent call out for us, not necessarily physical hangings, overdoses and things like you attend on an ambulance but we attended ones which sometimes involved chemicals or ones with access issues such as railway lines or water so that we could bring some added safety to the scene.

Until I was on HART, I attended hangings in private dwellings, overdoses by medications, as all did on the ambulances, but this was an eye opener seeing different types of suicide and how desperate people get.

We were tasked the one day, to a potential chemical suicide in Dudley. There is a famous pub there called the Crooked House. Look it up it really is an impressive building! To the back of the pub there is a large area of waste ground and we had reports that there was a male in a car who was unresponsive and had been found by a dog walker, which is normally the case.

We arrived at the location and pulled up about fifty metres away from the vehicle. I remember the vehicle make and colour still, and I remember it being parked up against some trees and not in a normal position if you were going for a walk etc. You start to notice things like this from the minute you turn up.

The Fire Service turned up to support us just after we arrived. We did not rush into the scene as it was reported that there were potential chemicals involved. On looking at the vehicle, there were danger symbols on the front and the side windows and another sign which said, 'chemical suicide, call the police'. This was a first for me and new for some of the lads. The male in the car from our position did not move and until we knew what chemical we were dealing with; we could not check.

Ed spoke with the FRS and it was decided that they would wear their breathing apparatus and go to conduct a 360 recce of the vehicle. Off they went and did a loop of the car and looked for any initial signs of life. They came back and reported that the chemical in question was helium which is a harmless gas when used correctly to blow up party balloons.

They cracked the doors of the vehicle and withdrew. They made it safe for us to approach once the vehicle had been ventilated. Mini and I were tasked to go and assess for signs of life or confirm death, which was more the likelier out the two. As we approached, we could see that there was a clear bag over the man's head with two black tubes running away from it. He was in a relaxed position with both of his hands still resting on the steering wheel. He was dressed in blue jeans and a black jumper and his vehicle was a mess with empty alcohol bottles scattered all over along with medication packets with his potential details on.

(D Team, back row left to right, me, Webby, Olly, front row Baarsy, Millie, Ed and Mini)

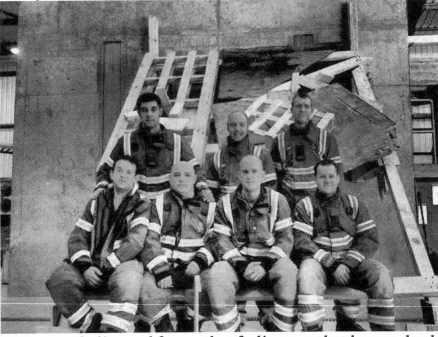

You get a feeling and for us, that feeling was that he was dead. We checked for a pulse on his wrist and neck. Nothing. There was no steam on the inside of the clear bag and no respiratory effort. He was cold and as always; we checked his legs where hypostasis was present. Unfortunately, he was long gone. This chap had got to a point in his life that was so bad he had made the decision to take his own life. What I find strange though still, is the time he took to print the signs for his vehicle to warn others and prevent them from being harmed. It is little things like this that stay with you. There is an element of kindness about it and a willingness not to harm others.

We looked at the equipment he used to take his life and it was a simple set up. He had a thick clear plastic bag on his head that had two back tubes running from it going to the rear of the vehicle. He had black tape around his neck to make a seal and two cylinders of helium in the rear of the car both with taps turned on. It looked like a failsafe to me, if one didn't work the other would!

You could tell he must have thought about this for some time and had made his mind up.

Sometimes with suicide you see a struggle or little things that tell you that death has not been instantaneous, like vomit or urine incontinence etc. There was none of that, he looked peaceful. He had to be around 40. He had an iPod around his neck and his earphones in. His eyes were shut already and as I said with both hands still on the steering wheel.

I said earlier you need to have a dark sense of humour as a paramedic, and I said to Mini.

"I wonder what he was listening too?"

Now this can seem a little morbid, but he was dead and there was nothing else we could have done for him; however, it is one of the little details that we try to piece together. I pressed the iPod, and the battery was just about to go but we saw that he was in fact listening to Bon Jovi soundtrack and the song was Always that was playing when we were with him. Obviously, every time I hear this now, I think of him.

This was a sad job but not one that really bothers me, it helps as I was in such a close-knit team, we debrief, and we move on.

CHAPTER 40

Social

We worked hard but we played harder as a team, we always made sure we would socialise as much as possible, especially at Christmas and for birthdays. One of Ed's fantastic ideas the one time was to do a 10-plate challenge at a local all you can eat buffet. It sounded a good idea at the time, it was not! Following a shift, we set off for a place called Cosmos and all you can eat buffet in Wolverhampton. It was standard stuff; we ordered a beer each grabbed a plate and started the challenge. There were a few rules and if your plate was not full enough then it would be referred to the plate committee for review. There certainly were a few suspect plates. There was curry, chips, vegetables, cheeses anything you could think of, it was not enjoyable in the slightest, but a challenge was a challenge. We were all throwing food down our necks like there was no tomorrow. Stupid, yes, but it was funny, in fact it was absolutely hilarious watching the lads gag and gip on their food and the staff looking at us with disgust. We looked like a load of lads on a stag do let alone health care professionals. It was great fun and crucial to our mental well-being. Team winddown and interaction was the key and reduced the mental health going into your rucksack. It stopped it from overflowing and getting out of control. Following the meal Mini was sick on the carpark, Olly sat in his car and wound the seat back to relax. No one won the challenge, and we were all ill for the next few days. Was it worth it? Of course, it was!

Rhoda and I had some amazing news. We were pregnant with our first child and could not have been happier. The jobs and exposure to the nasty side of life was taking its toll and we would see it on a regular basis on HART, but a job was coming up that really affected all involved and to this day it still does.

People ask me all the time these two horrendous questions.

"Did you ever kill anyone in the Army?" and "What's the worst thing you have ever seen as a paramedic?"

It is so hard to explain to people who are not in the job. Over the years I have seen some really disturbing things that no medication can ever take away. I believe some of these incidents are far worse than my military experiences. Incidents include dead children in RTCs who were not wearing seatbelts, kids who have drowned in outdoor rivers and swimming pools, their parents begging us to save them, an old couple who have died together in their armchairs due to a faulty boiler. I have delivered babies into the world that have been still born, hearing the cries of the mother as we tried so desperately to save their children. Parents who have physically shaken their babies to death as they could not deal with their cries, brutal murders that were committed by their own family members, suicides and holding someone's hand knowing they are going to die and I would be the last person on earth they would see or hear. It affects you, if it does not there is something seriously wrong with you. Over the years the death toll mounts up and it overtakes the actual good stories and the good outcomes you have with patients; it is a really tough job. The content of the next chapter I have never publicly spoken of, we attended an incident where following it, I had a big wobble, the rucksack overflowed and wanted to explain how it felt and affected me.

CHAPTER 41

<u>One bad job away from quitting</u>

On the 14th March 2012 Rhoda and I welcomed baby Logan into the world and from that day on everything changed. Rhoda did absolutely amazingly now we were a little family of three and I was a dad. I was delighted, holding my little man in my arms for the first time is truly special. We named him Logan due to our love of Wolverine from the X men. It was nine pm exactly when he was born and shortly after I was kicked out the hospital, they have tight security at New Cross in Wolverhampton, the same place I was born years before. It was a special evening, and I did not know what to do with myself. I called my parents who were over the moon, rang my friends, then just went home for a sleep. It was a long day and Rhoda felt the same too. Very traumatic a time but so special none the less and we are truly blessed and grateful that we had Logan in our lives.

This changed things for me without me realising. I had previously attended jobs involving children and although harrowing, I could brush it off and crack on with things, but this was about to change when I attended an incident that I cannot remove from memory.

It was Summer 2012 and Mini, and I were put on a relief shift with another team for nights. We turned up to station and no one was there, they must be out on a job. Ryan, our acting team leader for the night made contact with them and they said that they were on an incident in Herefordshire, reports of drowning. That is all we knew at that point, so we scrambled to get all our kit and personal protective equipment (PPE) together and to make our way in the reserve minibus to back the team on the ground up. Blue lights on, we flew down the motorway to the site of the incident, monitoring the situation as it started to unfold. The HART on the ground already had their brief and got ready to deploy. The report we had was that there was an adult male and a three-year-old child missing in a weir section of a river. This heightened our senses as with all jobs with children involved.

We arrived on scene and it was chaos, multiple fire crews in boats had been deployed, police cordons were in place. This was a big job. There were other assets on scene too Seven Area Rescue Association (SARA) who also had boats and operatives deployed. We got kitted up for working in swift water. Not the most comfortable gear but it was really good kit that would allow us to operate in water for some time. We had an all in one dry suit that took some getting into, boots and a personal flotation device (PFD) that would allow us to be tethered in the water so we would not be dragged down stream and of course medical equipment ready to treat any casualties.

Using our buddy-buddy approach we helped each other get into our PPE as quickly as possible to assist the other team, it sounds long winded but the call by this stage was only forty minutes old so the window to find the missing casualties was still alive.

We were briefed on the situation and it was good and bad news. A father had taken his family out on to the water to the rear of their property for some leisure time. In the boat there was the father, two kids aged around six and a child aged around three years old. It was believed that they had got into difficulty and went over the edge of a weir and were forced under water. Before anyone arrived on scene it was believed that the father managed to get the two older children to safety with the assistance of a brave policeman and local villager. One of the kids was in cardiac arrest and basic life support was given on site and subsequently they were transported to hospital. I believe they survived, thankfully, but that was no consolation to them.

It was then reported that the father who managed to pull his two kids to safety then ran back into the water to try and rescue the third and he was not seen again until later.

We were now on site, in the hot zone and the day crew were relieved and stood down from the operation. Lucy and I were tasked to cross the river and relieve other staff and await instruction to start the search again, we had Neil from SARA with us too.

Mini was tasked to work with the fire service on a boat downstream so that he could rapidly deploy to us if we had found either the father or the young child. Me Lucy and Neil were tasked to conduct an independent search of the sweepers and strainers (trees in the water) at the right side of the river. Before we entered the water, we could see the family's boat still washing around in the weir, fire crews trying desperately to free it. The water was so powerful, and it was like a washing machine, if you get dragged into a weir you are in serious trouble. We had to go into one on our training, attached to a rope and it was really scary. You are pulled underwater and then re-circulated, surfaced, and dragged back under. This is totally out of your control and that is why we feared the worst for this young lad and father who would have been so tired and helpless at this point.

We entered the water; it was around chest height; the water was really cold and we were probably about twenty metres away from the weir and still felt its full force. We were tethered by ropes and being supported by crews on land. We searched the side of the river, prodding our poles on the bottom to see if we could feel anything, we searched in between the overhanging branches and felt underwater just hoping to get hold of something.

As time went on that makes any realistic chance of survival

very unlikely however we had to consider the human factor on this. What I mean is, by this stage we had the mother of the family at the side of the river, watching everything that was going on. Sky news was on scene and with that added pressure we knew it was slowly turning from a rescue attempt to a body recovery, however we had to do the right thing.

We continued searching and light was starting to fade, we moved downstream a little further and Neil made the discovery. He had found a young child face down in a sweeper. Neil grabbed the child and passed him down the line to Lucy and then Lucy passed him on to me as I was closest to the riverbank. It was truly horrific, he was freezing cold, naked where his clothes had been ripped away by the currents of the weir, and he had bruises all over his body. He lay lifeless in my arms with eyes wide open and fixed, his little airway full of water. He was not breathing and had no pulses anywhere that I could feel. I wrapped him in my arms and got him out to dry land. It was obvious that this poor little child was dead, his long hair covered his face and eyes. I cannot forget this sight and doubt I ever will. We made in my mind the right decision to start resuscitating him. This in my opinion was the best decision. Why? If he is dead, then nothing else to do! It is not the way we do things. We were all aware that this child was dead however we resuscitated him for his onlooking mother, to show her that everything possible was done for him, but we did this for us too. Later down the line we would re live this nightmare and if we simply did nothing, for me it would not be closure. By doing everything in our power, despite knowing the outcome, is brave and makes us human. We commenced basic life support on the opposite side of the river. I was doing CPR and Lucy was ventilating his lungs. At this stage Mini was tasked to come and get him from us via boat to take him back to his mother and the Critical Care Team over at the other side who was set up ready to receive him.

Mini was at the side of the river, I picked up this little lad and continued to press on his chest until I reached my mate Mini. I passed him over and Mini continued to resuscitate him until he was in the care of the doctor.

They continued to do what they could but unfortunately the outcome we all knew was coming, did, and his death was sadly confirmed.

Staff welfare is excellent within HART and Ryan the acting team leader asked if we were ok to crack on and we were. We had given the mother some closure, but we all wanted to get her husband out too. He had been now missing for an exceedingly long time and light was now non-existent. By this time, Mini and I had swapped roles and he was in the water and I was now on a boat, he was prodding the ground with a pole and systematically covering the ground in a desperate attempt to find the father.

Mini could be a real irritant at times and he used to wind me up, I said before I could of strangled him at times, but do you know, in real times of need, he would bloody step up to the plate and do what he could to help others. It was around 22:00 and it was nearly time to call off the search. The staff were so committed to seeing this job through, the water was extremely cold and Mini must have been freezing by now. He felt something with a prod of his pole on the bottom of the riverbed.

"I think I've got him" He shouted to us.

We made our way over to him in the boat. The water was flowing hard and I could see Mini was tired. Still attached to a rope, Mini went under the water in an attempt to lift him off the deck. As he did, Mini and the body of the father came to the surface, at the same time Mini started to get dragged downstream by the current and the weight of the father's body. He was in trouble and perhaps should have let go of the father to look after himself. He did not! He hung on for dear life. We got a hold of his tether and pulled as hard as we could until they were both at the side of the boat. The two firefighters pulled them both into the boat. Mini was exhausted but he had done so well, unfortunately the father of this family was dead, he had lain on the riverbed for some time now. It must have been awful for him knowing he had saved two of his kids and had to go back for another knowing that they may never come out again. A really brave act and heart-breaking at the same time.

We had done our jobs as best we could, now was time to look after ourselves. Mini was hypothermic and we had to get him sorted quickly. We had a kind offer from a villager who said that we could use her hot tub to warm him up. We didn't take her up on the offer as it was not appropriate, instead we got his clothes off and warmed him up. He is one of these annoying buggers who does not drink hot brews, if there was a hot bottle of Coke, he would have been well away.

This job really affected me and maybe because we had just had Logan, maybe as it was so prolonged and I had so much time with the child, I cannot put my finger on it but years down the line I still see his face when I am sleeping and still get overprotective of my own kids when near water. This is due to years of pulling people out of locks and weirs. The human mind is really complex though, as this job really bothered me, but others did not.

We were awarded commendations for this job, which did not mean a thing, we were all only glad to do what we could and enable this family to get some closure.

CHAPTER 42

The Mental Struggle

I mentioned before about the rucksack on your back. Over the years it fills up with trauma and depending on how you process that trauma, depends where it ends up. Some of the trauma is dealt with at the scene of the incident, some you may think you have dealt with and it will come back to bite you in the arse. I had been a soldier and witnessed and engaged in some horrific things at a young age but thought I was ok. The drowning incident affected me more than I thought it would. This is when I started to notice changes.

The numb feeling went on for days and weeks to come, I would not be able to sleep properly. This then affected my mood and temperament to others. I would wake up in my sleep quite regularly now, would scream out, bed sheets would be soaked through with sweat and embarrassingly I occasionally pissed myself. What the hell was going on with me? Was it that one bad job? Or was it a culmination of everything? I later found out it was exactly that, a culmination of life experiences that were not yet processed in my mind.

Afghanistan was a problem, not due to my actions in killing or bearing witness to death of fellow soldiers, it was a fear of being killed myself. This heightened feeling of anxiety and living on the edge in Afghanistan, day in and day out came back to haunt me.

I started to have vivid flashback or dreams, whatever you want to call it. I would see a flash of light from an incoming object and then wake when it struck me, like those dreams you have when you fall and wake before you hit the ground. I would have dreams where I would be drowning and this young child would be alive and I just could not get to him, I would wake up exhausted. I knew that I was having issues but did not share them with colleagues or Rhoda. I would go to work and nobody would really know that I had anything major going on, I was happy go lucky, always the joker and I would get home and take it out on Rhoda and those close to me.

I was really struggling, and it went on and on in a vicious cycle. I would argue with Rhoda at home, blame her for things and just be nasty and my behaviour was awful. I would not admit that a former paratrooper and now paramedic would be suffering. Over time everything got worse and worse, I remember days I just sat at home in my underwear, staring into space, not being able to function as a normal human being. I felt low and worthless, no sense of duty or pride anymore.

I recall the one day taking all my military pictures off the wall at home and not wanting to see anything from those times. As time rolled on, I turned to alcohol and drank more than I should have which we all know is the worst thing to do. I would not talk to my partner Rhoda or friends I was shutting down.

I had a beautiful young lad to look after, and the sad reality was I had no interest at all in him. I felt ashamed and could not get myself out of this position. I started going sick from work and my character changed, I was selfish and had no feelings whatsoever, I thought of nothing or no one.

The lads in the team noticed a change in me and I started to get aggressive with them, bite their heads off over little things, make mountains out of molehills, there was no perspective or thought process in place for me.

The one day I remember us discussing things as a team around the incident and one of the lads said.

"We shouldn't have resuscitated that kid, he was dead"

Looking at it now, he had a point, from a clinical perspective we knew the outcome, I know that, but at the time in the frame of mind I was in, it was not what I wanted to hear. I stood up from my seat, picked the chair up that I was sat on and threw it right his way, it hit him and it was that moment I knew I was totally out of control and needed some help. What was I doing? This behaviour is not normal at all? I was not functioning properly, I was not eating or sleeping correctly, I was being horrible to the woman I love, I was doing nothing with my son. I got to that darkest point after all these things happened and thought, "What is the point in me being here?".

This frightened me but in my mind I was slowly convincing myself that life would be better for everyone else if I wasn't around, I am making Rhoda's life hell, my son Logan would be better off without me, I treated my team and mates like shit, they wouldn't miss me. This for anyone who has gone through a breakdown before will know all too well.

Mentally, I was fragile and, on the edge, from the outside looking in I had no reason to be unhappy, but for me I reached that point where I needed to make a decision.

Unfortunately, now it really upsets me to put this down on paper, but the decision I made was not the right one. I wanted to die, I did not want sympathy or was not crying for help, I was just that low, it felt the right thing to do. I would not admit that I was suffering, I blamed myself for the position I was in and wanted to end the pain. I was contributing nothing to my family, I was off work sick now and my mind was made up.

I was going to go for a walk to some woods in Codsall where we were living at the time and hang myself. The reason I thought about this was from my experience of finding people hanged personally. It would be a dog walker who I did not know who would find me, so they wouldn't care less and then my family would not have to see me. How bloody selfish was I to think it would not affect anyone?

Luckily, before I could do any of this, Rhoda, who I thought hated me by now, put some calls in to my GP and local services and started the ball rolling for me to get some help. Rhoda and I sat down for hours and I completely broke down, tears pouring down my face, I was telling her I did not want to be here anymore, and it all came out. She saved my life. Writing this now, I am so grateful for her support it must have been so hard to manage. I will forever be in her debt. From there I was lucky. I was treated by the GP and referred to specialist Veterans Mental Health Services. I had years of counselling, cognitive behavioural therapy (CBT), eye movement desensitisation and reprocessing (EMDR) which was really powerful and worked well. I was subsequently diagnosed with complex post-traumatic stress disorder (PTSD) by a clinical Psychologist and given years of treatment. I had to work really hard to get out of the mindset I had and to this day still struggle, but the coping mechanisms I have in place and the amazing support I have from my now wife Rhoda is a debt I can never repay.

I still take medications and will have to for the rest of my life but every day now I looked to be positive and push forward and do good rather than slip back to those dark times I had. My advice for anyone who is struggling, for whatever reason, is just to simply talk, get things off your chest.

CHAPTER 43

Final Moments

With my wobble under a certain amount of control I felt in a good place again, a weight had been lifted off my shoulders and I was keen to push on in my career and do as much as I could for my patients.

HART was probably the best three years I had on the job so far, I was part of a fantastic team, we got to attend the best jobs but there was often no hands-on medical treatment. I missed that side of it and wanted to do more and more. It is a very surreal feeling when you are on the ground in an ambulance at an RTC for example, in the middle of nowhere with just your crewmate dealing with a critically injured patient or patients. Dealing with the noise, confusion, screaming or silent patients, getting on the radio to summon help, doing the basics really well and trying to save life, you are making a difference just by being there and telling the patient they are going to be ok holding their hand and just giving that reassuring voice in their ear.

Sometimes it turns out well and other times not. On many occasions I have been the very last person someone has seen or heard before they succumb to their illness or injuries and I am very privileged to have had that honour.

I recall one night it was pouring down with rain it was around 11pm and I was working on the RRV and was sent to RTC near

Spaghetti Junction, Birmingham. It came through as an RTC entrapment and when I arrived, I nearly missed the incident as I could not see through the windscreen due to the rain. I was flagged over by a member of the public. A car had skidded off the road and into a concrete pillar that held the motorway up. There was no one around which was not normal, just me the lady in the vehicle and a kind chap that had stopped. The vehicle was crushed like an accordion. I took a few seconds to way up the scene and requested back up from a Trauma Doctor and I requested to make ambulances 1, I asked for the Fire Service and the Police through or EOC.

I grabbed my equipment from the rear of my vehicle at the same time asking this very shaken up witness to update me on what happened.

"She must have hit that wall about 100 mph mate, I heard her screaming but I couldn't go over, sorry mate, I was worried I just called you" he informed me.

At this time, the screams were really distressing, and this man was really upset.

"Mate you have done a great job, we will get her sorted thank you, go and sit in your car in the dry for a minute". I said to him.

As I got closer to the car, I started to see the full scale of the situation. All the front end was crushed up to where the steering wheel should have been, the driver's side window was smashed and all I could see of this trapped lady was an arm and the side of her head. She was mechanically trapped, and it was clear I had no way to get her out on my own. Within minutes, comprehensive screams of "help me!" were turning to muffled sounds and I knew she was in big trouble. It was dark and all I had was the light from the front of my car, I reached in through a 30 x 30 cm gap and put my hand on the side of her face and then down to her neck and grabbed a pulse. She had a rapid pulse that was quite thready, and I could feel her chest area was cool and clammy, just from this I knew she was in shock. I felt down to where her legs should have been and everything was deformed, my blue nitrile glove now covered with bright red warm blood.

All these checks were done rapidly but I felt helpless, she was in end stage hypovolemic shock. She was trapped she was losing her airway. I could not see anything, all I could do at that stage was give her some intramuscular morphine sulphate to ease her pain, hold her face and her arm and reassure her that I was there with her. She must have been so frightened and by the time I had got to her the coherent screams for help stopped and the noise of an insecure airway started. I had no way to monitor her other than a basic pulse check and airway sound. Eventually the snoring was unbearable, and I managed to find my way to her mouth and push a super glottic airway device (IGEL) into her mouth and down her airway to secure it as best I could. She was unconscious now else she would not have tolerated it. I did what I could and could now hear that the fire service was just pulling up behind me. I knew it was too late, but we had to keep going.

A white helmet appeared by my side and asked,

"What do you need mate?"

I replied, "She needs to be out now, she's trapped and going to arrest any second".

The fire service worked like lightning to free this young woman and I had to stay by her and comfort whilst the lads and lasses from the fire service cut, spread and smashed their way into the wreck of this vehicle.

The damage was that bad that twenty minutes had passed and by now we had a doctor and an ambulance on scene to support me. The police were chatting to the witness and this was a proper multi agency job now all pushing in the right direction to save this woman.

We set up a stretcher and gathered our advanced life support equipment and were ready to go as soon as they had freed her.

She was finally now out of the wreckage, her lower limbs were angulated, and blood covered from head to toe and with an airway sticking out of her mouth we set to work. By this time, she had catastrophic bleeding from her lower limbs, tourniquets were applied to both legs, her airway was secured with the IGel I inserted earlier. We cut through her clothes and got to her chest, she was not breathing and no pulse. We attached the defib pads and assessed that she was in asystole, which means no cardiac activity and we commenced CPR. The doctor was at the head end and the crews and I got to work on this traumatic cardiac arrest. So, without going to deeply into the process, we had to do certain things during a traumatic arrest than a normal medical one. We had to quickly assess for reversible courses of the arrest, Hypoxia (deprivation of oxygen) Hypothermia (Temperature), Hyperkalaemia (blood toxicity) Hypovolaemia (Blood loss) clearly present and the four other causes, Thrombosis (Clots), Tamponade (Pressure on the wall of the heart), Toxins (Poison) and Tension pneumothorax (air trapped in the plural cavity of the lungs.

Now, some of these we could not do much about at the roadside, but we did try to reverse the ones we could. For her blood loss we used an intraosseous needle and drilled a hole into the top of her arm which allowed us to push fluid back into her system in an attempt to manage her blood loss, we did this via a three-way tap, large syringe and two litres of sodium chloride. Her core temperature was managed with blankets and foil wrapping at the roadside and due to her chest trauma, we attempted to rule out a tension pneumothorax within her lungs by decompressing her chest. In this process we would use a large bore cannula (needle) find our landmarks which was the second intercostal space, mid clavicular line. We pierced her skin above her third rib and pushed the needle through to her lungs to decompress her lungs on both sides. You would hope during this brutal procedure that you would her air or see bubbles on the end of your cannula to confirm it had been successful, I am afraid this was not the case. Blood came back up both tubes and it was clear her chest cavity was full of blood. We were coming up to twenty minutes of resuscitation on this young women, looking around everyone was focussed and working hard to prevent the inevitable, blue lights flashed around the stone pillars under the M6 motorway, there was a tube in the woman's mouth, blood on the floor and on everyone's hands and despite all our very best of efforts, she was dead. The trauma was just too much. Twenty minutes up and the doctor called it, she was confirmed dead. Following this call there is a real sombre moment where all the noise seems to stop and we as colleagues look at each other and say.

"You ok? good job mate".

We knew we did everything we could. We gave the women some dignity after inflicting even more trauma on her in the driving rain at the roadside. We covered her up and started to make our kit up and tidy up, this is then the start of reflection. We handed the scene over to the police and headed back for a brew and a chat, this is all that is needed at that point, a few hugs too, and to chat through what we had done. The most privileged part for me was at the very start. I was the very last person on this earth that she had heard, and I was the very last person to put my hands on her to comfort her, a stranger, that was a privilege. I never found out her name until it came out in the newspapers days later. I do not know if she had family or loved ones, but one thing I know is that I will never forget her.

CHAPTER 44

From land to air

The best of the best in my opinion were those red angels who landed next to you on an incident in an EC135 helicopter, helped you treat the most severely injured patients and then whip them off for further care at 200 mph in the ambulance of the skies.

These were the men and women of HEMS, (Helicopter Emergency Medical Service) of the Midlands Air Ambulance Charity. Working on this highly prestigious service was the pinnacle of any ambulanceman or women's career. They have the best training, equipment and only go to the most serious of incidents. To work on HEMS you need to be a little special, but I for one was a little short on confidence and never thought that one day I would be able to wear that red flight suit and become and air ambulance paramedic.

I recall Weave and I were on a job once and exactly that happened as mentioned above. We were called to a nasty RTC and then we heard the unmistakable sound of the EC135 coming into land. The crew were amazing, really professional and engaged with us. They were real team players and at the time I was an EMT, I said to Weave.

"Wouldn't you want to do that mate?"

His response was always the same.

"No do I fuck!" He does make me laugh.

Weave was one of the best paramedics I have ever worked with, but his outlook was literally to turn up do the job as best he could and go home for a few beers. I could not find fault with this outlook at all.

I had now worked on HART for around two and half years and had got to know some of the HEMS crews quite well. One of them asked me why I had not applied before and I just said that it was a confidence thing. I knew I was a good paramedic, but I did not think I was in that higher level. Luckily in my team at HART, Baarsy was previously a HEMS crewmember, well back when the Wright brothers invented flight anyway, and Olly was current, so I had chance to pick their brains. I looked up to them both of them and they both had loads of experience and both were clinically very knowledgeable. The bonus of being on HART was the time we had to train. With their help I made sure I was clued up on the trauma side of the job and brushed up on the medical side. The lads gave me the confidence to at least apply for the role when it came up which is what I was going to do.

The time came and there were six vacancies for part time HEMS crewmember roles across the region. I was up for it and applied on NHS Jobs and the wait began to see if I had made the shortlist. This was the first recruitment in years and was open to all applicants internally and externally from West Midlands Ambulance Service. There would be hundreds of candidates who would apply and from that six would get the positions. The odds were very low, but I did get comfort of the fact there were so many applicants and many of whom would fall at the first hurdle. I had nothing to lose but my biggest fear was looking like a failure or embarrassing myself in front of those very same HEMS crew who I had got to know over the years. I prepared myself for the challenge. The good news was that I had made the shortlist and was invited to attend a HEMS selection day. This was known to be the toughest of selections in the ambulance world and I wanted to get it right.

Such was the demand for the positions there had to be two

separate selection days. There were sixty on the first day and sixty on my day, like I said the odds for me were not looking great.

Over the years my bad back had been a real problem for me. I believe it all had stemmed from my young soldiering days and exacerbated over my time as a paramedic. I knew there would be a physical aspect of the selection process and knew I would have to ignore the pain if I wanted to shine through on the day.

We arrived at RAF Cosford the home of Helimed 03 where we would complete our recruitment day. I looked around and there were some familiar faces of paramedics with whom I had worked previously, and I felt beaten already. I had worked with some of these guys and girls before and to their credit, I knew how brilliant they were. I refocused and looked at the areas in which I could outshine them and try to implement the plan.

The day would consist of a physical and mental test along with some clinical scenarios, which were the ones I was worried about most. Not due to going through them, the fact they would be assessed by people who I knew and wanted to impress.

The first test was a mile and half run around the whole perimeter of RAF Cosford. I knew I was fit, but also had a back niggle, this would be time to put on paratrooper mode and just fight through. I knew that I would have to complete the course quickly but also be a good team member too, it was not about 'check me out look how fast I am', it was about supporting others and not belittling them at the same time.

We set off and I was tucked in the middle, the grey man as they say, and I saw a tall chap bomb off like lightning. It was big Steve Mason, he was rapid and clearly was an ex-soldier like me, you can just tell. I thought to myself, he is going for this I need to keep on his tail. I ran as hard and as fast as I could to catch him but no matter how hard I pushed, that gap remained the same. Everyone I ran past I gave encouragement to, as Steve did, and we entered the last four hundred metres. There was no way I could catch him. I saw him finish and with true team spirit he turned and cheered me in.

"Come on, push,"

I gave it all and finished strongly. I came in second and together Steve and I ran back to support others who had given their all. This was not for show, this is clearly who we were, the military had taught us to support others which we did.

One event down, it was now time to hit the gym and go through the RAF fitness test.

This test was a best effort, how many press-ups and sit-ups you could perform in two minutes and then followed the dreaded bleep test, last man or woman standing. You may be thinking at this point why do you need to be this fit to work on HEMS? The simple answer is that potentially you would have to land two miles away of an incident and carry all your emergency equipment on foot, over fences, gates and through the streets to get where you needed to be.

Off we went banging out the reps, paired up with a buddy, pushing each other on, you could see in all their faces who wanted it and who did not.

I smashed the press-ups and sit-ups and now it was down to the bleep test. Levels 1 to 5 most of the candidates were there or there about. Following this level, people started to drop, left right and Chelsea. Once again, big Steve and I were the last men standing and the competition was on; but not for long, I was hanging out and the better man won.

Physical assessments done, it was time for lunch, a quick chat, and the final assessments of the afternoon. Ahead of us now was a maths exam, and a medical and trauma assessment. I felt confident in the fitness and OK about the scenarios but maths, I was dreading. It is no joke I am a paramedic, but absolutely shocking at maths. I administer drugs that could potentially kill you if not done correctly. Maths and being a paramedic do not go hand in hand I assure you. We have set, ridged guidelines to help, and with muscle memory and a book in my pocket at all times, I have never had an issue. So please do not let it put you off, a little work and you can pass if you want it enough.

I went into the exam and the questions were out of this world.

I do not believe Stephen Hawking could answer half of them. The bit where I came into my own in the numerical exam was the map reading section including the use of grids. This was basic compared to dropping artillery on to someone's head in Afghanistan and the need to be precise or people died, basic six figure grids was all it was.

I knew that I had dropped points in the maths exam and was prepared for this. Any other day this would have bothered me, but I knew I would have to shine in my medical and trauma scenarios if I was to stand a chance.

I need to thank Olly. He sure did put some time in with me on the scenarios, people do get really put off by them as they are not true to life in many respects, however you need to show a process throughout. I find if I talked through mine, with actions, that was the best way to get through, but practice is key.

I had a scenario that a farmer had been impaled on tractor spikes on a rural farm in the middle of nowhere. I arrived in the air ambulance and off I went through the drill. I followed CABCDE, Catastrophic haemorrhage, Airway, Breathing, Circulation, Disability and Environment. At each point on the ladder going into a full and methodical assessment. If I found anything, correct it, and reassess. It sounds simple, but in front of your peers, it was hard going. I was more worried about looking more of a nob than normal in front of them.

I felt I did well and proceeded on to my medical scenario. This was the same again, a lot of basic paramedic assessment skills, with a difficult ECG (electrocardiogram) to break down at the end. It was tough and it took me a while to get what was going on as ECGs are not my strong point, but we got there.

It was a long day and I felt I did well. I shone in the physical side and prayed that I did enough in the rest. I spoke to a few candidates and they were more confident than me, but as with everything, we would have to wait to get the call, come to interview or thanks for attending but...

A few days went by and I was back at HART doing my normal stuff and bumped into a few of the HEMS lot who were on our assessment day,

I asked, "well then? come on you know what's the craic, did I do ok?"

"We can't say anything Dave, we all had to promise!"

I thought you buggers! They bloody know too! The only thing they said was that I did very well and was up there around the top candidates. I took comfort from this and knew if that was the case, I had done myself proud.

The call came. I shouldn't have felt so negative, but I couldn't see out of all those good people there I would get through to the next stage. I was too self-critical because I had done enough, the Air Ops Manager said,

"Dave you did really well mate, we would like to invite you through to the next stage, formal interview".

I was not expecting it, but I tell you what, I was fair chuffed, it was now time to clue myself up to the max on the EC135 and the Midlands Air Ambulance Charity.

Interview day arrived, and the interview panel included Ian Roberts (Air Ops Manager) and Ian Jones (Aircrew Manager) and a woman from HR. I dressed as smart as a carrot again and got ready to wow them with my knowledge. I was prepared for a formal interview, but it felt quite relaxed. I answered all their questions, giving examples when appropriate. I spat out all I knew about the charity, how much it cost to run three aircraft, where the bases where etc. I felt confident in my delivery. Historically, some aircrew had a bad reputation for pissing off the ground crews. I had never experienced this myself, only the good side. But Ian Jones asked a question and I could not believe the answer I gave back. "What would you bring to the Midlands Air Ambulance?" he asked.

I replied, "Great work ethic, willingness to learn, good morale for the troops and the ability not to piss the crews off!"

Oh dear that one slipped out!

I was asked by HR if I had any criminal convictions, I said, sadly yes, went on to explain the circumstances and one of the panel said,

"Work hard play hard".

When it came to my military career and colourful past, they were non-judgemental, and the interview was wrapped up. I shook all their hands and left.

I had done all I could and now it was up to them, if I had somehow done enough to become a HEMS Crewmember it would be my biggest achievement against the odds. I would become elite in the pre- hospital care world and be on top of my game.

I felt chilled and Rhoda, Logan and I were plodding around the house one day and I remember looking out the window to the back garden when the phone went. It was an unknown number and I answered,

"Hello "

"Hello, Dave, its Ian Roberts"

"Oh, Hi Ian, how you are doing?" acting as if I wasn't expecting a call.

"Good thanks mate, just want to say thanks for attending the selection day and interview, you did really well mate",

I thought yeah, I know what's coming next.

"We would love it if you would come and join us at the Midlands Air Ambulance Charity".

I can honestly say I was ecstatic, writing this now I can feel the butterflies in my chest. I had made it! Out of all those great candidates they saw something in me that they liked and wanted me to be part of their team.

I got off the phone.

"Well? "Rhoda asked.

"I'm in "I said.

She gave me a massive hug and said I knew you would do it; she was so proud of me which meant the world to me.

Training for my new role was about to start. Originally, I was a little naughty as the HART Ops Manager at the time said that he would not be able to support anyone from HART who applied to HEMS on a part time basis. There were two of us from HART who were successful, so I chose to leave and return to Willenhall on the ambulances as I wanted to be on HEMS so much. I had a fantastic three years with the mighty lads from D Team, but I could not pass up this opportunity.

Big Steve Mason had passed, my mate Pete Edwards who I knew from back in the day had made it, Lozzy from HART was on and the final two were Kelly Bennett and Mike Smythe, all these men and women were absolutely fantastic. We were the six that made the cut.

We started our intense HEMS Crewmember course and we learnt all things from the theory on air law, focussing on the Air Navigation Law, mission definitions and emergency checklists, detailed training on meteorology (weather), navigation, principles of flight, aero medicine and crew resource management.

This was a really testing course, but I could not have been with a more supportive team, it was amazing. Hands on learning with an EC135 sat right outside the door.

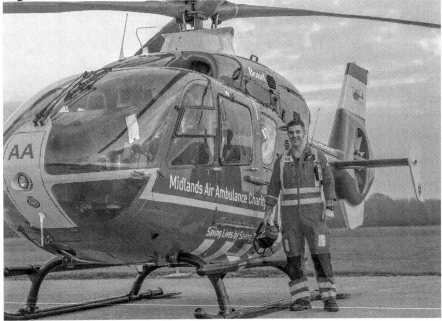

(Me and G-EMMA)

Also included on our course was the ground handling aspects, simulated exercises, loading and unloading aircraft safety and fire training and safety checks. The highlight of the two weeks of course was the flying. We all had three practise flights, lasting 1 hr 15 total covering an initial familiarisation flight and a navigation line check to ensure that we could become a fully qualified HEMS Crewmember. It was bloody tough and not much time to have a jolly and look out the window of the aircraft, full on navigation and drills.

The course was very much like doing your driving test, you pass it, then you really start to learn. Our HEMS journeys were just about to begin.

Big Steve Mason had passed, my mate Pete Edwards who I knew from back in the day had made it, Lozzy from HART was on and the final two were Kelly Bennett and Mike Smythe, all of these men and women were absolute fantastic, we were the six that made the cut.

We started our intense HEMS Crewmember course and we learnt all things from the theory on air law, focussing on the Air Navigation Law, mission definitions and emergency checklists, detailed training on meteorology (weather), navigation, principles of flight, aero medicine and crew resource management.

This was a really testing course, but I couldn't have been with a more supportive team, it was amazing. Hands on learning with an EC135 sat right outside the door.

Also included on our course was the ground handling aspects, simulated exercises, loading and unloading, aircraft safety and fire training and safety checks. The highlight of the two weeks of course was the flying. We all had 3 practise flights, lasting 1 hr 15 total covering an initial familiarisation flight and a navigation line check to ensure that we could become a fully qualified HEMS Crewmember. It was bloody tough and not much time to have a jolly and look out the window of the aircraft, full on navigation and drills.

The course was very much like doing your driving test, you pass it, then you really start to learn, our HEMS journeys were just about to begin.

CHAPTER 45

Potato Hill

Pete and I were going to be based at Tatenhill Airfield in Staffordshire or Potato Hill as we fondly called it. We would be part of Helimed 09's aircrew. Tatenhill was a beautiful place, a World War 2 training base that was built in 1941 just outside Burton and right next door to St Georges Park, home to England Football.

It was a really friendly and welcoming base and it felt like home. It had a family atmosphere and was run with real fluidity with Ian Jones at the helm, or Scooby as he was better known. We had a well set up portacabin with the hanger for the aircraft just outside. In the summer months you could see all sorts of private aircraft taking off from the runways and even got to see a few VIPs now and then dropping into the England camp. I felt so proud to be part of this unit.

Our pride and joy would be G-EMAA (Gemma) she was a Euro-copter EC135 and she would get us in and out of HEMS scenes with ease. She was a twin-engine light utility helicopter and was capable with a speed of 161 mph or 200 mph with the wind up your arse. Charity donation funded at the cost of £4.5 million and a cost of £25 pound per minute to run. The MAA run three aircraft to serve the public and day after day they are making a difference, saving lives by saving time.

On the base we had two full time pilots: Matt and Chris. They were both absolutely fantastic and they could not do enough to support us. I do not know if it was fate or not, but it turned out that me, Pete and Matt all attended the same high school; Great Wyrley High School, but at different times, and when crewed together we were affectionately known as the "Wyrley Bird", I bet none of our teachers saw this happening. Chris was a former paramedic before becoming a pilot and understood both sides of the coin. Both lads were really approachable people as well as fantastic professional pilots who took us under their wings, literally, when we first started.

A daily routine on a HEMS shift would run the same day in and out, it was not rushed, and certain checks had to be done to ensure safety and as long as we booked on our start time, all was good.

Aircrew on a shift would consist of a pilot and two HEMS Crew members, to start with I was on with Scooby for my first few shifts. What Scooby did not know about the aircraft or being a HEMS Paramedic was not worth knowing. He was the most knowledgeable mentor I think I have ever had. As with every relationship we had our difference of opinion, but I believe we made a great team, and I was keen as mustard to learn as much as I could from him. We would all turn up in a morning, first one there opens up and puts the kettle on. That was me! Then we would get changed into our super tight red flight suits ready for the day. Medical equipment was next, bags checked and then we would sign out our individual drugs which at the time was 20 mgs of Morphine Sulphate along with Diazemuls, Oramorph and Diazepam. We also had an RRV at the base that needed checking just in case the weather was rubbish and we had to respond by vehicle. Whilst this was going on the pilot would be in the hanger, checking the aircraft, testing the fuel to make sure there is no water in it, and prepping the aircraft ready to get out onto the pan. Once they have completed their checks in the hanger, they start the aircraft and fly it out the hanger! Only joking they do not really! They must use a bit of kit called the

Heli- Lift which grabs the skids of the aircraft and lifts it off the ground. Simply then, the pilot guides it with ease into the position he wants it and we are all set.

As a crew you do everything together, cleaning, simple maintenance, assist with start-up checks, navigation and re fulling. There was lots to think about and do but I must say it was a great team to be in with everyone knowing their role inside and out.

We would then grab our brews then go and sit with our Captain for the met briefing. This would ensure we were all briefed on the weather, hazards, for example gliders or fireworks and anything else of relevance for that day. We were trained to read Terminal Aerodrome Forecast (TAF) and METAR which is a weather observation, and NOTAM, (notice to airman). I wish I could give you an example of these, but it would take me to the end of the story to explain it to you properly.

Fully briefed it was time to book online with the fabulous team who sit on the Airdesk at EOC, wish them a good morning and then go into daily routine.

I would love to say sit down and have a brew, but in twelve hours there was always something to do. Training, aircraft washing, practicing missions, kit familiarisation and of course to make time for base visits for members of the public and friends of the charity. Once again, I felt really privileged to be part of this charity and the highlight for me was to come.

A few days had passed on my first stint on the Air Ambulance, and I didn't want to wish an injury on anyone, but we hadn't turned a wheel. We had taken the aircraft in and out for my first three days. Granted, I did loads of training and familiarisation, however I had not completed one mission. I was a little disappointed, but I would get my chance.

The next set of shifts arrived. It was in summer and the weather was fantastic. I would be busy, I thought, and I was not wrong. I remember my very first HEMS job: I was on with Scooby and Chris for the day and my role that day was to be the treating paramedic, so I would be travelling in the back. This meant that when the red phone went on station, Scooby would answer it and get all the details such as type of incident, grid and location, then he would make his way to the front seat and start prepping the map and inputting grids onto the aircraft system. The job came through as an RTC entrapment in a little village just outside Lichfield, not far away from us at all. It sounded pretty serious and as well as us attending we would be joined by HMED 03 from Cosford which had a doctor on board. It was my first HEMS mission and inside I was buzzing and, as always, calm on the exterior. I had to do the basics and that would be enough.

We grabbed our helmets and walked out towards the aircraft. Chris and Scooby jumped in and started their checks, and I was stood outside the front ready to complete the first part of my role and assist with the aircraft start-up.

There are two engines that need to be started and it was my job to make sure there was no one incoming who could be hurt, and to check there is no fire on start up. As you look at the helicopter the right side is number one engine, the left is number two. Dependant on what day it was, odd or even would depend which one the pilot fired up first.

On this day it was number one. Chris put one finger in the air, (not his middle one, although he did this a few times) which told me that I need to move to the right side of the aircraft and monitor engine one. My reply to acknowledge him was one finger back - simples.

You can hear the jet fire up and the blades slowly start to turn. The smell of that ever-familiar jet A1 fuel shooting up the nostrils took me straight back to Afghanistan. With the blades gathering pace, Chris now pops up two fingers to me, palms facing luckily, this was the signal for me to move to the number two engine side and monitor the same.

With both engines now idling, I get the thumbs up from Chris, to enter the disk and board the helicopter via the sliding door at the side. I plugged in my headset or else the noise would have blocked out any conversations that happen so I can chat freely to them both. Scooby would now assist Chris with the pre-flight checks, and it would be my role to update EOC via radio that we were mobilised and to give a rough ETA. The pre take-off checks were vital and were a challenge and response cross check to ensure everything for flight was ready. An example of a few from Scooby to Chris would be "fuel cap?", "key check", "autopilot?", "on, upper modes set", "engine main switches?", "Flight, gated". That last one was my personal favourite as you can hear and feel the engines going from idle to flight, the power, noise and vibration increases, and we are almost set to depart. The gated part means that the flight switch once pushed upward to flight has a gate that goes across it so it cannot be tampered with whilst in flight. It would be a little awkward if it dropped down mid mission.

The last checks would be security to make sure all the doors were locked, and seatbelts fastened, then Chris would give a quick brief to us as to how we would leave the base, i.e., a runway departure and a direction.

We were airborne, and it felt good getting my first start up completed. I let EOC know that we were airborne, and ETA was around ten minutes. There was absolutely no time to take in the scenery this time, we were soon in the overhead and could spot the blue flashing lights of an ambulance and a fire appliance already on scene. We could spot the vehicle that had clearly rolled several times off the narrow road into a nearby field. We conducted an orbit of the scene and between us three decided on a safe place to land, obviously giving some considerations to the terrain, slope, any overhead wires and access to the job itself, everyone has a say in the matter and if one person is not happy, it does not happen. Luckily, this time we could land really close to the scene as it was an open field with no obstructions. As with pre take-off we had to complete arrival checks of similar fashion, safety is paramount for us and for everyone else underneath us.

We came in nice and steady and once committed, kept quiet to allow Chris to put down safely. Once down with the rotors still running, we had to wait for Chris to give us the 'clear, go.' At that point, I would grab the two bags from the stretcher, dump them at the side of the aircraft, let Chris know I'm going, wait for his thumb up, and head off toward the job. Scooby did the same and we were on scene. From receiving the call to landing the aircraft was literally minutes, checks and verifications seem pretty long winded, but everything is done in a timely manner.

We got a quick brief from the team already in attendance and set to work. We walked over to the vehicle which was severely damaged and had clearly rolled multiple times, dirt and debris was everywhere. I could see a male still hanging upside down from his seatbelt but trapped by his door and the steering column. The paramedic crew that was already there were doing a good job of trying to manage him whilst still in a difficult position, he clearly had a reduced consciousness level which was concerning. We got closer and I could smell alcohol on the man.

Now we could hear the sound of Helimed 03 inbound, and it was pretty certain that we would need the skills of the doctor on this one. The patient was incoherent and combative at points. He clearly had a head injury but until freed, we would not know the extent of any other injuries he had.

The fire service worked hard and nearly had him out. We had to consider this patient's mechanism of injury of course but we were more concerned about him losing his airway at the time.

As the other aircraft set down next to ours in the field, we planned that this patient would need a Rapid Sequence Induction (RSI) on scene. RSI in its simplest form is putting someone to sleep to better manage their airway and behaviour management.

It is a process whereby there is an identifiable need to manage the patient, for example, in this case, it was a head injury with associated poly trauma with a risk of aspiration. Once the patient was freed by the fire service, we had already set up an RSI station. We had an ambulance stretcher next to the vehicle with a scoop stretcher on it, we ensured a good 360-degree access and all the equipment needed to complete the procedure. Some of this included monitoring equipment, suction, airways and oxygen, plan B kit if anything goes wrong with plan A.

Now the doctor was on scene with us he managed the scene overall but once the patient was on the stretcher it was up to us to perform a rapid assessment on the gentleman and rectify any immediate threats to life from catastrophic bleeding, his airway, breathing and circulation. We identified that he was bleeding from his lower legs and had bi-later tibia and fibula, compound fractures, however there was no catastrophic bleeding at this point. His airway was patent and self-maintained, he was breathing on his own, however it was very rapid and would need more diagnostics on the secondary survey. Circulation was present, and he had a rapid radial (wrist) pulse. His disability or neurological signs were alarming. Glasgow Coma Scale (GCS) is what we use to assess someone's neurological capacity. It is measured out of 15 which is me now as I am writing and is the best response. The lowest score would be three and that would mean that someone is totally unresponsive. It is measured through behaviour, eyes opening response, best verbal response, best motor response which are all scored appropriately. A score of eight or less as the saying goes, GCS under 8, intubate, but believe me this can be misinterpreted.

Our patient, following our initial assessment, scored eight out of fifteen. His eyes were open spontaneously which is a four, his best verbal response was incomprehensible sounds, a two and his best motor response was abnormal extension of his limbs, also a two.

We applied our monitoring equipment which read his oxygen saturations, ECG, and blood pressure, along with CO_2 in preparation for the RSI.

Everyone agreed as to what needed to be done. He needed to be knocked out and flown to a major trauma centre and get a scan done to the lay person.

Everyone had roles, one was airway, another monitoring, the doctor was in charge of administering drugs, the fire service would fetch and carry (not to be disrespectful to them) and the final stage before anything happens is the checklist read out by the doctor to ensure everything is ready. You are literally stopping someone breathing, in a field in the middle of nowhere, it needed to be done right. All immediate life-threatening issues were taken care of and we set about managing this patient. Time now for the 6 Ps: plan, position, pre-oxygenate, prepare, paralyse, post intubation. This simply means that we would deliver as much oxygen to the patient via a mask, we would then sedate the patient to a point they stop breathing, paralyze their vocal cords to allow us to place a breathing tube down their trachea to allow us to effectively breath for them and this would then allow us to better manage them and get them to a definitive place of care quickly.

Now ventilated and controlled, we went to work on his legs, pulling them both straight and aligning his sticking out bones as best we could and assisted loading him onto the doctor's aircraft.

Job done and a great team effort. It has been doom and gloom in parts but for every bad experience I have had, there are better, and this was one of those. A few months later, I got to meet this man who we had a part in helping and, had it not of been for the actions of all involved, he would have died. He was having a rough spell and had a drinking problem, but following this, he had cleaned himself up and re-connected with his young family and made a better life for himself. I take pride in my small contribution.

We made up our kit and got ready to return to base. By this point, a large group of people were all swan-necking over the fence with their camera phones trying to catch a peek at someone else's misfortune. This is something that made my blood boil! Some would help, but others are much more inclined to stand over you, recording someone who is having the worst day of their lives so that they can update their Facebook profile and get some likes! It is outrageous.

When we lift out of a HEMS scene, there are a couple of ways we can do this, dependant on the terrain and the surroundings. People ask us:

"Why do you take off backwards?"

"Why do you go really high vertically before setting off?"

These are very good questions, but it is simple. We sometimes lift from the ground and fly up and backwards just in case we had an engine fail, that would then mean we could follow the same path back down to the ground knowing it was safe on the way in. Certain times, we fly really high before we set off and in similar fashion this could be due to being in a built-up area and do not have the room to go backwards but the same rules apply. It is all safety and when you are flying in and around buildings and cruising as low as 600 ft safety is paramount.

The jobs kept rolling in now and I got some great experience dealing with critically injured patients. The added extra of course was flying to jobs in an aircraft and landing in some really diverse places. I recall the one day I was up flying with Matt towards Shropshire and we could see a massive rain cloud just in front of us which would have brought visibility down to zero. I was also on with Ivan at the time and we needed to look for a place to land. We searched for a safe landing site and we soon spotted one.

"Anyone need anything from Sainsburys?" I asked over the internal radio. "That will do us" Matt replied.

We looked down and Sainsburys in Telford had a massive car park that was completely empty as luck would have it due to the store being closed for maintenance. We can normally land in a 40 x 40 metered square area, the size of a tennis court, so this was plenty.

The challenge was now on for Matt to land in a parking space - no pressure Matt! The car park had no hazards such as wires or loose debris, fresh tarmac on the ground so it was perfect. We came into land and underneath us I could see the white lines of a car park space. We set down and Matt absolutely nailed it, inch perfect and just before the rain came down. We were safely on the deck and over the radio I heard:

"Go on then Dave".

"Go on then what? "I replied.

"Go and get a ticket, we aren't on a job, so we need to pay our way".

Fair enough I thought, and I opened the side door and jumped out, took a wander over to the pay and display machine and dropped a quid in. We had an hour's parking. Ivan and Matt were laughing as I climbed back in and stuck the ticket to the window. This was a bit of morale boosting after all, and of course, we never heard the last of how good Matt's parking was! Over time, I became more and more confident in my clinical abilities and was a good crew member. The clinicians I had round me were the best of the best and they had the same drive and commitment to helping others as I did. It was mentally exhausting at times, especially in the summer when you were out all day and only returning to base to refuel. The clinical exposure was greater than that I had experienced before, but the downside was that you were dealing with lots of young kids, sometimes in the most horrific of circumstances. I recall landing at a job, and once again heard the screams of a parent who had survived the RTC, and her child was being resuscitated by a crew at the side of the road when we arrived. It was so traumatic for her but for the crews too, you cannot remove things like this from memory but what you can do is be a good human being and try your best to help.

Tragic accidents were something I was more accustomed to by now and the one time, we responded to a report of a child drowning, but not one like I had experienced on the river when part of HART, but in the child's back garden. You must be thinking how could this happen? but tragedy it happens all the time. This job was in a private dwelling around the Tamworth area, and I recall landing in a field some way away from the actual job and the police picked Walley and I up and drove us on blue lights to the property a couple of minutes up the road. We could not land safely anywhere closer. We knew it was a two-year-old, but we had to remain calm and not let that influence our safety and that of others when it came to picking a suitable landing site.

We ran into the address and we were told that the child's dad was looking after him and cleaning the windows at the back of the house but was unaware the child had fallen into the fishing pond and got caught under the netting and subsequently drowned. When the father climbed down from the ladder to check on his son, he was met with a sight that would haunt him forever. I get chills just writing this now. How would I feel if it happened to one of mine? Everyone on scene again was doing everything they could for this child. A decision was made for us to continue resus and get this kiddie to the best place which would be Birmingham Children's Hospital (BCH) I radioed back to the pilot on the aircraft, who was not our normal pilot but thankfully had experience of landing into BCH and updated him that we would need to get into BCH asap with a patient and his father.

Once again, we had to make quick decisions, this child had to be resuscitated, that was fact, the father had to come with us, fact, reality was that the chances of this child coming back was slim, however drowning is a funny thing and there was still a chance. We stabilised as best we could with basic CPR. There is absolutely no time to fanny about with anything other than that at the time. The next issue was that we would not all be able to go in the aircraft with the child. The fuel limits on the aircraft meant that we had to be a certain weight to lift from scene, this unfortunately meant leaving Walley behind on this occasion, but he ensured that we had a quick start up and departure from the site to the hospital. Walley gave our EOC the heads up and they informed the hospital that we were inbound using the ATMIST method, age, of patient, time of incident, mechanism of injury, injures seen or suspected, signs and observations, blood pressure, GCS pulse that sort of thing and treatment given, along with an ETA.

With lots of moving parts and lots to think of. Not only was my job to continue to resuscitate this child, but we also had to make best decisions on time frames, options on treatment, would it have been better to go by land on an ambulance, do we leave dad, risks and benefits and you have to make good decisions in the most difficult of situations. This kid was dead, and we all did what we thought was best. From the point of call to me loading onto the aircraft with the father and child was around thirty minutes. The first resource arrived and started CPR after seven mins following on from the father trying desperately to do it himself.

Not only did I have to look after his child, but the father too. He was numb, vacant, and hopeless. I had to get Walley to lead him to the aircraft and physically strap him in as he was incapable at the time of functioning. He needed to see everything I was trying to do to save his son.

We approached the hospital, which is another nightmare, you are coming into Birmingham city centre and had to fly in between buildings and land on the main road just outside the hospital which thankfully the police had shut for us. I shouted across to the patient's father,

"You sit there and don't move until I come back to get you!"

He did not acknowledge me.

"Do you hear what I am saying?" I said to him again and he nodded.

The reason for this was that we needed to keep the rotors running in case of a breakdown, we would have shut the whole city. We were well versed and practiced in this, but it needed good communication and control from me and the pilot.

We landed on and I got ready to run out and deliver this child to the medical team who were waiting just outside of the building. I asked the pilot if I was clear, he replied "clear, go" I scooped up this poor little kid who I had been desperately trying to save and legged it about twenty-five metres as fast as I could with him, placed him on a stretcher and the team jumped straight in and went to work whilst moving back into the hospital. I had to run back to the aircraft, with the rotors running, that familiar smell of the fuel, with everyone in the office buildings watching out the windows. I got the thumbs up from the captain and I ran under the disc to get dad. I had undone his belt and made sure everything I had used in the back was secure and doors locked. Thumbs up again I led the father by his arm away from the aircraft and into the care of a nurse who was waiting. The aircraft now had to lift and go to a secondary site where he would wait for me to return.

I went into the resus room and everything that could be done was being done. A doctor came over to me for a handover whilst his team went to work. He listened to what I had to say, the treatment I had given, timings etc and he was supportive of our efforts.

They resuscitated him for a further hour, but it was no good. I completed my paperwork and went to pass on my condolences to the father. I tapped him on the shoulder and said.

"I am so sorry mate; we all did everything we could".

With tears in his eyes, and still feeling numb his reply was simply.

"I know".

His life had just changed forever in the space of little over than an hour and he had lost his son and would probably blame himself forever. I felt distraught for him.

It is no lie that I shed a tear on the way back round to the aircraft, I was gutted for him. Another job for the rucksack that I will have until my dying day. It was not every shift things like this to happen but for sure they are the ones you remember.

CHAPTER 46

Captain Fantastic

I was so fortunate to work alongside some amazing people on my time on the aircraft some of whom I now call friends. One to mention in particular is Captain Chris Levey. He is an absolute gentleman and would really give James Bond a run for his money when it came to turn on the charm. He is a real professional who would always do his very best for his crews and muck in with the best of them. Ivor, Chris and I were at Potato Hill one shift and we had chance to cook some breakfast, comprising of bacon, eggs, and sausages - all low calorie of course. The conversations were down in the gutter as normal and banter was flying around the crew room until Chris had a bite of his sausage cob, or bap or balm whatever you want to call it. I said something ridiculous as normal, and he started to laugh.

We were all laughing but Chris stood up and made a weird noise. Ivor and I laughed even more as we thought he was taking the piss. As it turns out he was choking on a sausage! It took a while for Ivor and I to really get with the programme. We knew it was serious when we looked at his eyes, the fear in them was genuine and his body language suggested he was in trouble. He walked into the kitchen area of the crew room and by this stage was noticeably quiet. Ivor and me to the rescue! He could not cough, breathe, fart or anything! This sausage was properly stuck. Both of us big men, Ivor and I took it in turns to wallop him as hard as we could between his two shoulder blades in an attempt to dislodge this bit of sausage. Seconds later a bit of sausage shot into the sink and he started to make a better noise. I bet he really scared himself! I know I would have been worried, but he was in the right place. Two Air Ambulance paramedics to the rescue and our glorious Captain was breathing once more. Tears rolling down his face and a couple of seconds to catch his breath and he was back in the zone. What a legend! We laughed it off, without eating at the same time and cracked on. Funny now, but not at the time.

Over the years though, choking had been no laughing matter. I had been to old ladies in nursing homes killed by a digestive biscuit. Kids choking on grapes, (always make sure you cut them in half) I have pulled steak out of people's airways too! It is amazing that, within a blink of the eye, it could all be over. We all had a fantastic relationship on base and I loved every second I was there. I felt really privileged to be part of the Midlands Air Ambulance charity, even if it was only part time. I had fulfilled my ambitions and got further than I could have ever imagined. We had managed to save patients' lives and make that difference and that is all you can hope to do.

The stresses of the role were always there and to this day, some of the amazing people who I got to work alongside are still there doing the same job day in and out, witnessing horrors and doing their absolute best in the toughest of roles. As my partner, Rhoda was still a paramedic and we had our little lad Logan to look after, it put a definite strain on things and the Air Ambulance work was very unsociable at times. From where we lived, I had to commute an hour, complete a 12-hour shift then commute back, sometimes five days a week. Although it was worth it, was a pretty full-on lifestyle. The bonus was that Rhoda understood, she was a shoulder to cry on and my only really support and to this day I am so grateful to have her at my side.

I had a run of a few bad jobs on the aircraft and seemed to have a run of one unders. This is how we describe suicides by train. Not a very nice way to go but for whatever the reason, people do make up their minds that this is how best to deal with things. I had been to jobs where one man actually tied his dog to the track just before putting his head to the line and ending it. I really felt sorry for him as this was how desperate he was, but at the same time I remember feeling angry and disgusted that we had to deal with his headless dog afterwards, which upset more staff than the man on the line did. I remember talking to the driver following this one, and he said that he saw the dog tied down and the man tried to move out the way before the impact however, he was not quick enough. I feel for the drivers who, through no fault of their own, had to witness this.

I recall going to a job where a male had jumped off a platform in front of a high speed West Coast Mainline train and by the time we landed, he was dead but stuck on one of the front buffers.

All of these were definitely horrendous sights, but worse was to come when we had to remove him by using a jiggly saw to cut through his torso and peel him off piece by piece and pop him in a body bag, as the British Transport Police said they could not. The jiggly saw cut through him like butter, all his organs, still warm dropping out on the rails in front of us with one of the policemen trying not to gag and hold a clinical waste bag under it. The smell was horrendous, but if you ask any ambulance staff, over the years you get used it and I can honestly all the smells - death, vomit, shit and piss, I never gagged once. Like I said earlier, everyone who works on the frontline, police, fire or ambulance will see true horror over time and yes, war was horrendous, but it was very different, and my old colleagues have their own stories.

CHAPTER 47

<u>The last flight,</u>
<u>Stand down</u>

R hoda and I had made our minds up that we wanted to uproot and move up north. We wanted another child and we loved the idea of moving closer to the Lake District. It was in a place called Troutbeck, Cumbria where we found out we were pregnant with Logan whilst on holiday and loved the idea of relocating.

It was my last ever shift at Tatenhill and it would be one to remember, not in a good way though. I was working with Lozzy and that was a real treat as we had trained together and it a nice way to round things off. We were going to go for a meal after shift and have a few beers so that we could all get together as the Potato Hill family, staff, and friends of and have a good send of for me. it was nice that they had planned this for me, it was a sad time, but it was the right thing for Rhoda and I to do at the time and I have no regrets. I said it would be one to remember, but not in a good way, here is why. We booked on as normal, got the aircraft ready to go and were ready for the call. A call came but it was from the Air Ops Manager. I asked if everything was ok as I could hear she sounded different.

"I am afraid that I have some bad news".

This didn't sound good at all. Unfortunately, she went on to explain that one of our Air Ambulance colleagues was dead and she wanted to let us know. I cannot go into too much detail, but we were all devastated. We were all struck numb and between us, we decided that we would have to come off duty for a short time to take in what had happened. We discussed between ourselves what we thought had happened and eventually the detail came out that our colleague had taken their own life. There are stories of the reasons why, but I do not want to go into any detail. This news was absolutely tragic, and it shook us to the core. I wish I could say this was uncommon in the emergency service world, but it is not, I know now of six people. For my last day on the aircraft was one to remember, I did not want to go for a beer, it did not seem the right thing to do at all, but the team decided to go ahead, but the mood was horrendous. People were just sitting there and putting on a brave face and saying nice things to me, but it did not sit right with me at all. Granted, there was nothing we could have done, but it just felt awkward, and we were all very sad. I did get some lovely presents but looking at them now still remind me of our friend and colleague and that will forever be the case. We raised a glass and that is all I can say on that one as I do not wish to upset anyone with what I write. Our colleague was such a great person who shall always be missed.

CHAPTER 48

<u>Grim Up North</u>

I applied for a job with North West Ambulance Service (NWAS) and was invited to Liverpool for interview. The interview was very informal, but I will always remember one of the interviewers who was flicking through my personal development folder and saying.

"Oh, so you have been on the Air Ambulance and Hart, I bet you think your something".

Wow! I thought where did that bloody statement come from?

" Are you feeling ok? That's a little way off the mark, I am here as advertised for the job of Paramedic". I replied to them.

This boiled my blood a little bit and the other two who were interviewing nodded their head in appreciation. I basically shut up this gob-shite with a chip on her shoulder! I knew I had done OK as I had everything they needed on paper. My attitude was spot on and my feet have always remained on the ground. I had no time for Tommy Two Shits or Gerald who could bench press five cars if you could only do four! Unfortunately, people like this were everywhere. I came from the military and had respect for everyone I ever came in to contact with, however, you give it the big one and you would soon be brought down a level. I could deal with aggression and violence from patients, they may be ill or under the influence, but I would deal with that in an appropriate manner. I would not wind people up to make myself feel good and believe me there are people also like that out there, who normally end up crying about it. Respect is key and it must be earned, and I should once again be starting from the bottom with a new service.

Before I started, once again my criminal past had to be brought up and before I was given a job offer. An Operations Manager had to approve the convictions to allow me to work at his station.

Luckily for me, Mick Mayfield who was the Ops Manager was a Navy Veteran of the Falklands conflict and he had my back. I was off to Lancaster Ambulance station. I was now a normal paramedic back on an ambulance and started out to work in my new area. The staff up north were amazing, really accepting of me and welcomed me with open arms. It was a different way of working up north, different type of ambulance, different protocols but same old job. Same type of patients, the good, bad, and downright ugly, same smells but one thing for sure was different, the pace of life.

Northerners are mega, they call a spade a spaaaaaaaade, tell you how it is and are horizontal in everything. Everything is 'be rite', and 'grand as owt' I loved the station, staff and the whole experience of living there.

I remember my first meeting with Mick. I sat down in his office.

"Welcome Dave, I will make you a deal". He said to me.

"Go on then". I returned.

"If you keep shit I have to deal with off my computer, I will go above and beyond to make sure your right"

I loved him already, he had been there and done it, got the t-shirt and had the respect of everybody. You shit on mick at your peril. He was a hard-faced bastard with a heart of gold and a man I would have followed over the trenches for sure.

I made sure I just did what I had to do and cracked on. The job for me now was same old on an ambulance and living the high paced life on HART and HEMS was no more. It started to feel like just a job again. The usual mix of chest pains, piss heads, and of course, the odd nasty thrown in, to which of course I gave my all, but felt I still had one more exciting role in me.

I had done lots of following in my career so far and had leadership experience in battle and from a clinical position as a paramedic but I wanted to lead people again, empower them to be better clinicians, utilise my experience to help them flourish. I had learnt from so many amazing people over the years, Alistair, Weave, my team on HART and HEMS and felt at this stage of my career I had made an impact on my patients but now wanted to help others the way I had been helped previously. The same pattern of jobs followed me from the midlands up to the north, from chest pains to baby delivery, RTCs to cardiac arrests. All in a day's work for a paramedic. A comedy moment for me in my time up north, although not funny at all for the patient at the time was as follows.

Steve Barton and I were sent to a bungalow for a concern for welfare job. Now, this type of job meant that they were either dead, on the floor and can't get up, or done a runner in the night. We arrived, met the nosy neighbour, "His curtains ain't been open for two days, six hours and fifty-two minutes, twenty seconds," They know it all.

We banged the door.

"Hello ambulance, anyone in?" we called.

Nothing. We looked for any windows that were open, but we couldn't see through the curtains, and it was now time to break the door down.

With a slight nudge we got in the back door without any damage or noise. The place smelt damp and the house was very untidy with shit everywhere. Sometimes, you would find someone dead in bed, hanging or just simply out. We got to the bedroom and saw a pair of mottled legs coming from under a wardrobe that had obviously fell on top of the patient.

At first glance we thought that he was dead. There was no sound, no movement. We would get the wardrobe off him to see what was what. As we lifted the furniture up, we could see he had no clothes on, but were amazed at the size of his......well you know.

I said, "Jesus look at the size of his...."

Before I could get the rest out the man under the cupboard said.

"Never mind me cock, get this bastard cupboard of me!"

We shit ourselves, thinking he was dead, and he could here every bloody word.

"Sorry old pal be with you in a minute".

There is quite a lot of poverty up north and in my three years with NWAS I went to more suicides than I did previously in all my time in the midlands. These casualties were mostly men aged from eighteen up to around sixty years of age, but something I had never experienced up to now was a woman that had done the same.

I was on the RRV at Morecambe station and I had a call for a female hanging and it threw me completely, I had never done one of these before. As an experienced clinician I was really apprehensive and did not know what to expect.

I pulled up outside the property, neighbour met me outside and said,

"She's dead mate".

I walked inside this bungalow which was a beautiful property, clean, fresh and tidy, but as soon as I took a look to the left, there she was, a woman in her fifties partially hanging from a ladder with her toes just touching the floor. The ladder was coming out the loft and she had used really thin para cord and wrapped it tightly around her neck. I do not know why it affected me so much, was it because she was a woman and I hadn't experienced it before, I do not know but I got to that point again when the rucksack was filling up again once more.

CHAPTER 49

<u>Leadership</u>

I f I asked twenty people what makes a good leader, I would get potentially twenty different answers. I think that is a good thing especially in the roles I have been in, but I feel that leaders do need to have certain qualities to put them in that position, that said I believe everyone has the power to lead. What I did over the years is look at certain people and think, "bloody hell, he did that well, or look how he reacted in that situation". If someone asked me to do something would I do it? Do I respect them enough, or is it an order?

I was lucky enough to work with a pilot called Chris Whip. This was a small world moment, but he had been a pilot of an Apache attack helicopter the very same time I was in Afghanistan. He had flown missions to support us in Sangin and now was flying me in and out of HEMS sites. We started talking one day about leadership and the difference from the military and civilian life and at the time he had just finished writing his book called The Leadership Secret. It is an amazing book that I would highly recommend. It does not teach you how to become a good leader, but it does give good examples of practice and over the years I had picked up my own style collected over the years working alongside good leaders.

Leading men in a firefight was one thing, they all had the

same training, values, and professional foresight to help you out. In the Ambulance Service you had people from all walks of life, backgrounds, sexuality, beliefs and do you know what that meant to me? absolutely nothing. I would firstly treat each and every colleague, patient as I would want to be treated myself, with respect and dignity. 99.9% of the time, there would be no issues but some people you just would not be able to connect with, and that's fine, just as long as you engage with them in an appropriate way. Yes, people fall out, say things they don't mean in haste or when upset, stressed or going through hard times, but as long there is understanding, or an apology if needed, then happy days.

For me, and in my opinion, a leader should have good qualities without negative. There was now an opportunity for me to become a Senior Paramedic Team Leader, (SPTL) with NWAS. It was a clinical supervisor role with up to ten clinicians in your team, from new starters to old hands and would require a flexible individual leadership approach to get the best outcomes for all.

I applied for an acting role to test the water and then for the full role following that. I had been with NWAS for around a year now at this point, so people knew me and I them. I had to move from Lancaster station further around Morecambe bay to work from Ulverston, Barrow and Millom stations. I finally had my team, and they were a great, dynamic bunch. Many personalities and experience levels but as earlier, I just kept my core values and leadership style at the forefront of my mind. This is not the definitive model for leadership, but it is mine, here are a few qualities I believe kept me on the right track.

Honestly, I believe you need to be completely transparent in front of your team and peers have no hidden agenda and be able to answer truthfully anything that I am asked. This is the same when dealing with patients and difficult scenarios, honesty is the best policy. Be up front, do not hide anything and if you ever make a mistake as we all do, be honest it will work out much better.

Competence, I believe this is essential in leadership, you cannot expect your staff to do their best and maintain a high level of care if their line manager cannot do the same. It was important to me that I get out with my team, do the same as they did, maintain high standards and show good practise. There is nothing worse than an incompetent leader, it will reduce morale and impact on the relationship.

Communication is key, we all have different issues that are ongoing, we may be in different stages of our careers, some may be happy in their role and some not so it is essential to communicate effectively with everyone in your team. Have an open-door policy, give me a call but this said, you need to ensure you have time for yourself as not to get overloaded, share the burden with your seniors if you need. Communication is normally the first thing to break down in any situation.

Experience, some people say it counts for nothing, but I have to disagree, for example over the years now I have worked in many roles from the very first rung on the ladder to the top of clinical practice. I have dealt with many different types of incident from the basic to the major and all give you some experience. Now it is not about me telling a new starter, you have to do it like this or that, it's about me imparting my knowledge on to them so they can think how they would have dealt with it. This is how I learnt with the aid of debriefing following an incident, not to point the finger, get learning points out of it, we always want to improve in everything we do.

Character, for me is essential and you have to be one. You do not have to be a comedian and try to impress all the time, but as a leader you have to know a time and place for humour, empathy, praise, advice or debriefing it is a real balance and if you are not a character and robotic in all you do it will not work.

Lastly you need a sense of humour, my time in the military, the ambulance service, and the rugby club you need to smile. The job is hard enough at times so smile, be happy and have a laugh. When the time is right you can have a really good laugh. Weave, D team and I used to laugh all shift but when the job needed doing, we did it right first time, every time. People who are inappropriate or no common sense make me worry and it can get very awkward at times.

These traits served me well and I never had a bad experience with my team, does that make me a perfect leader? Certainly not, but it allowed me to work in a unit with different people with a common aim to get things done. I respected them and they me and we had a good time doing it together for the good of our patients.

CHAPTER 50

<u>18 years of hurt</u>

I n a period of around 18 years, I had fought on the front
line in Iraq as an 18-year-old lad. In 2006 in Afghanistan,
I had directly taken the life of others, seen my brothers in
arms die in front of me, and avoided death myself on a number of occasions, from then on, I had been on the front line of
two NHS ambulance trusts. I did my absolute best to save lives
and had many successes, unfortunately these are the ones that
do not stay with you. It is the men, women, and children that
I was unable to save that will haunt me to the day I die. This
is just my experience but, every single person who has fought
in war will have the same experience, every single person who
has been on the frontline as an NHS worker will have the same
experience, so I am not alone. Everyone has a story to tell, and
they all have had moments of elation and moments of distress,
heartache, and horror. My demons and my illness came from
my time in Sangin, 2006, I thought I was going to die every day.
That anxiety and feeling has followed me throughout the years
and I just covered it up with a different mask. Paramedic mask,
Friend mask, Daddy mask, until such a point you deal with your
demons. It is a lonely place but I am so lucky to have crossed
paths with so many amazing people in my time and it has been a
real privilege to have had these opportunities.

I have messed up so many times, I have hurt people physically and paid the price, I have hurt people who I hold close, and they still support me. Mentally I have been fragile and wanted to end it all, but I am still here. For all those mistakes and regrets I hope I have made up for them, I asked for help when I needed it, and held out my hand for others when they did.

I have been part and still part of the best brotherhood there has been, the, Airborne forces, a brotherhood like no other. I have my parents who still love me despite all the hurt I have given them over the years. Blessed with a brother, nans and grandads, aunts, and uncles, friends, and most of all, now a wife, Rhoda and three beautiful boys. They are my absolute everything and I would go through Afghanistan one hundred more times to make sure they are ok.

I have been so fortunate and had opportunities so far to kayak in Greenland with my mate, learn to ski in Colorado with the Not Forgotten Association and made friends for life. Rhoda and I went to the garden party at Buckingham Palace. Without the things that have happened to me, none of these opportunities would have come up and I am truly thankful and grateful to all who have supported me.

To give back I very much enjoy challenging myself and raising money for charity. As I mentioned earlier, Weave and I cycled from John O'Groats to Land's End in seven days raising money for Pilgrim Bandits Charity. I organised charity rugby matches and ran marathons all to give a little back. I will continue to do this for as long as I can so that these amazing charities can help others.

My faith in humanity over the years has been restored, there are some truly amazing people in this world and by me helping others gives me such a feeling of worth and accomplishment and that alone is payment enough.

I remember going out to see a WW2 Veteran, who was riddled with cancer, he had no friends no family and was dying. I entered his home, shook his hand firmly and said

"hello sir, my name is Dave"

"nice to meet you Dave, I'm Bill "he said as he gently gave my hand a squeeze. We chatted away for about an hour until his final words on this earth, I shall never forget this moment.

"Dave, I have to go now" he sighed

"Ok Bill, you rest easy now" and with that his eyes closed, his head rested back, and he drifted off peacefully. I placed my monitor on him and held his hand until there was no longer any electrical activity.

No friends, no family and just a good neighbour that was worried about him, if she had not made the call, he would have died alone.

What an absolute privilege to share Bills last moments.

CHAPTER 51

<u>Team Bentley</u>

I have not mentioned my family much as I wanted to save it for this point. Rhoda and I had Logan in 2012 and we had George in 2016 and this was also the year I married the most amazing women I have ever met. Rhoda saved my life and had it not been for her intervention, I would have been dead. I owe her my life. She is my best friend, my rock and support network that has stood by my side though the good and the bad times. She has supported me, understood me, loved me, and advised me from my lowest lows to my highest highs. She is so selfless she always puts me and the boys first and I cannot still believe she said she would marry me.

I proposed to Rhoda on Tower Bridge in London, we were first in the queue and I dragged her up to the glass platform and dropped onto my knee, she probably only said yes at the time as she is scared of heights.

We were married on the 5th of July 2017 at the Broadoaks Hotel near Windermere in the Lake District in front of close family and friends. Weave was and still is my best man and although we are miles apart, we are always true in heart. He looked after me so well when I was new, advised me when I was being an idiot, and if I asked, he would help me hide a body. To this day, a true friend and an amazing man that I can always rely on. We cycled the length of the country together in 2015, John O'Groats to Land's End, so if we handled 850 miles of each other and sore stinky bridges day in and out, we can handle anything. It was an amazing wedding, but it went so fast, we had our close family there and some great friends, too many to mention, but they have supported us always.

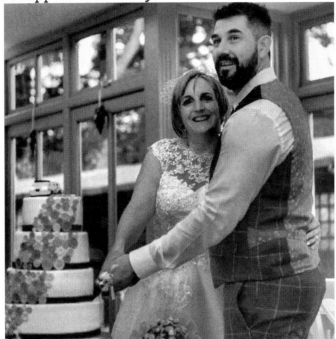

(Me and Rhoda on our wedding day)

We now have Jude who was born in 2018 and we have enough to make up the front three of the England Rugby Team, if they turn out to be rubbish, they can play for Scotland as their mum is Scottish.

We live in a little village just outside Lancaster called Bolton Le Sands and have some amazing friends here. We miss our parents every day, but the fresh northern air seems to do us good.

My body caught up with me eventually and my back now has so much metal in holding it together, years of abuse in the military and on the ambulance, service took its toll. We love the free open space and have our two smelly dogs, Albert and Pepper to look after.

Family is everything to me and after 18 years on the front line I decided to hang it all up for now and move in a different direction.

I love rugby, it is my sport and remember back at the start I said it saved my life, well now, I get to put back into the game. I love in my new role.

CHAPTER 52

RFU Injured Players Foundation

My new title is Injured Player, Welfare Officer (IPWO) and I left NWAS in 2019 to work in rugby. I know work for the RFU Injured Players Foundation who are England Rugby's official charity.

As the charity we support rugby players who have sustained catastrophic spinal cord injury or traumatic brain injury whilst taking part in rugby activity in England.

I manage the immediate welfare support for newly injured rugby players. I am the first person on the ground when their lives have been turned upside down and myself and our small team make sure they are looked after.

When the job came up, I could not turn away. I love medicine, I love rugby and the most important thing for me, I love helping people.

The people we support are truly amazing and I liken them to my friends who were injured in battle. They do not sit and sulk, they push on in life and have such a resilience and team spirit still despite sustaining their injuries it is truly humbling to be part of.

I get to host them at Twickenham in the injured players box, have a beer with them and watch the game, but on the other side work with Caroline who is my line manager and occupational therapist to ensure they have all the provision and care they need.

It is not as full on and frenetic as front line ambulance work, but it is just as rewarding. I utilise my communication skills and medical background to good effect and love the small team I am in at the moment. It allows me to have more time with my family and does not involve attending such traumatic incidents as before.

I would never say never about returning to hands-on medical practise, but at the moment I feel I am making a difference to other people and they rely on me just as much to support them as others did in their time of need.

The highlight for me so far was being able to run the London marathon alongside two inspirational injured rugby players, Dani and Ross. This is a moment I will never forget lapping up the real team spirit and encompassing all the core values of rugby. I look forward to doing the very same again in 2021.

EPILOGUE

This is a snapshot of my life so far, I wanted to share some of my experiences with you. I did not start out well and have made many mistakes along the way. I have been right, and I have been wrong. I have taken life but have also saved it. I have broken the law and paid the price; I have let people down who are closest and been as low as anyone can go. I have pushed forward and addressed my demons.

I have had the honour like no other to walk alongside true heroes and legends, witnessed heroism and bravery in the face of adversity, have been the last person there with a complete stranger in their final moments and have experienced things that I never thought possible. Out of it all, I believe I have become a better person for it. I thank you for coming along on my journey so far. Go out there and never give up follow your dreams.

Let me tell you something you already know, the world ain't all sunshine's and rainbows, it is a very mean and nasty place, and I don't care how tough you are, it beat you to your knees and keep you there permanently if you let it. You, me, or nobody is gonna hit as hard as life, but it ain't about how hard you hit, it's about how hard you can get hit and keep moving forward, how much you can take and keep moving forward, that's how winning is done. (Rocky Balboa)

DEDICATION

I want to dedicate this book to my wife, Rhoda, three boys, Logan, George, and Jude. I love you all so much, words cannot describe what you all mean to me and thank you so much for your love and support.

To my parents Glennis and Ben Bentley, I hope that I have done you proud. Thank you for all you have done and still do for me

to all my friends and colleagues in West Midlands Ambulance Service, Hazardous Area Response Team, Midlands Air Ambulance Charity, North West Ambulance Service. You all give everything still, selflessly to help others in need, you are all heroes and it was an honour to work with you.

Finally, I want to dedicate this book to all who have served and still serve in our armed forces, their families, and friends.

To those who never came home from our tour, Iraq 2003, Afghanistan 2006, we will never forget you and the ultimate sacrifice you paid with your lives. I hope we did you proud and that we still make you proud now.

Till the final RV in Valhalla R.I.P

They shall grow old, as we that are left grow old

Age shall not weary them, nor the years condemn

At the going down of the sun and in the morning

We will remember them.

(My beautiful family)

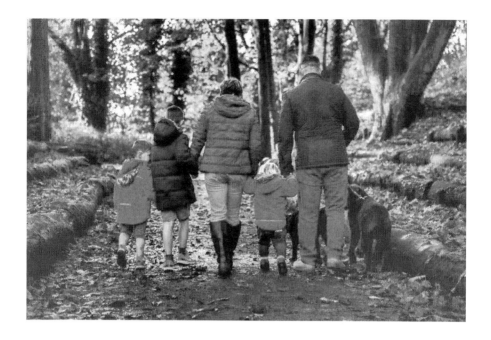

SPECIAL THANKS

Dan Hipgrave BA

Paul Humphries (Aircraft / Rugby photos)

Aileen Smith (cover)

Oliver Lee (Cover)

Pilgrim Bandits Charity

The Not Forgotten Association

Printed in Great Britain
by Amazon

59665885R00158